Practical Guide to Hereditary Breast and Ovarian Cancer III

Tomohiko Ohta • Hiroji Iwata • Nao Suzuki
Editors

Practical Guide to Hereditary Breast and Ovarian Cancer III

Annual Meeting of the Japanese Organization of Hereditary Breast and Ovarian Cancer 2023

Springer

Editors
Tomohiko Ohta
Department of Translational Oncology
St. Marianna University Graduate School of Medicine
Kawasaki, Kanagawa, Japan

Hiroji Iwata
Department of Breast Oncology
Aichi Cancer Center Hospital
Nagoya, Aichi, Japan

Nao Suzuki
Department of Obstetrics and Gynecology
St. Marianna University School of Medicine
Kawasaki, Kanagawa, Japan

ISBN 978-981-96-6778-9 ISBN 978-981-96-6779-6 (eBook)
https://doi.org/10.1007/978-981-96-6779-6

This Springer imprint is published by the registered company Springer Nature Singapore Pte Ltd.
The registered company address is: 152 Beach Road, #21-01/04 Gateway East, Singapore 189721, Singapore

Foreword

This Year Book summarizes the topics presented at the 3rd Annual Meeting of the Japanese Organization of Hereditary Breast and Ovarian Cancer held in 2023. The following are some of the medical and scientific topics related to hereditary breast and ovarian cancer (HBOC) covered in this publication:

One of the key highlights includes an in-depth explanation of the process from the discovery of BRCA1/2 genes to advancements in precision medicine and applications to public health. Basic science discussions cover mechanisms of resistance acquisition in BRCA1/2-related tumors against platinum-based therapies and poly (ADP-ribose) polymerase (PARP) inhibitors, as well as the role of BRCA1 in repairing estrogen-induced DNA damage.

Clinically, this Year Book addresses issues such as the radiation sensitivity of HBOC-related breast cancer, variations in age of onset, and risk assessment and management of HBOC-related esophageal, cholangio, and gastric cancer. Recent issues in preimplantation genetic testing for BRCA1/2 and other HBOC-related genes, including their implications and ethical considerations in Japan, are also discussed.

Furthermore, topics include the maintenance of genomic integrity mediated by DNA damage-related RNA-binding proteins (RBP), and the broader social and medical challenges related to the heritability of HBOC.

Additionally, this publication includes a "Statement from a Patient," offering valuable insights from the perspective of those directly affected by HBOC. The role of personalized care in improving patient outcomes and the latest trends in precision medicine are also highlighted.

Each chapter is authored by renowned specialists, making this publication a valuable resource for those involved in the management of HBOC, ovarian cancer, breast cancer, and other HBOC-related cancers. The information presented here not only aids in clinical practice but also supports the formulation of policies for improved healthcare delivery.

I would like to express my deep gratitude to Drs. Tomohiko Ota, Hiroharu Iwata, and Nao Suzuki for their significant contributions to the editing of this book. Their dedication and expertise have been instrumental in making this publication comprehensive and authoritative.

Tokyo, Japan
November 2024

Daisuke Aoki
Chair of Editorial Board

Contents

Part I
Basic Science

Chapter 1
BRCA1: An Enzyme That Protects Women from Breast and Ovarian Cancers: Revisiting the Evidence for Its E3 Ubiquitin Ligase Activity

Tomohiko Ohta and Naoe Nihira

Abstract The breast and ovarian cancer susceptibility gene product BRCA1 maintains genome stability mainly through homologous recombination repair (HR) functions against DNA breaks. While failure of this function causes carcinogenesis, it is also important as a target for treatment with poly (ADP-ribose) polymerase (PARP) inhibitors that induce synthetic lethality with the HR deficiency. In variants of unknown significance (VUSs), the HR capacity has been analyzed as a functional assessment to predict the risk of developing cancer. Thus, the assessment of HR function in BRCA1 is important for both carcinogenesis prediction and therapy. Pathological missense mutations in BRCA1 are concentrated in the N-terminal RING finger domain and the C-terminal BRCT domain. The RING finger of BRCA1, together with its structurally similar partner BARD1, forms a RING heterodimer with E3 ubiquitin ligase activity. Since its discovery more than 20 years ago, the biological and clinical significance of this enzyme activity has gradually become clear. In this chapter, the authors describe what is currently known about the E3 activity of BRCA1, which is important for carcinogenesis and PARP inhibitor sensitivity.

Keywords BRCA1 · Ubiquitin · E3 ligase · Homologous recombination · PARP inhibitor

---

T. Ohta (✉) · N. Nihira
Department of Translational Oncology, St. Marianna University Graduate School of Medicine, Kawasaki, Kanagawa, Japan
e-mail: to@marianna-u.ac.jp

T. Ohta et al. (eds.), *Practical Guide to Hereditary Breast and Ovarian Cancer III*, https://doi.org/10.1007/978-981-96-6779-6_1

1.1 Introduction

BRCA1 has multiple biological functions that contribute to the maintenance of genomic stability, but the HR function of BRCA1 is generally considered to be most important for its cancer-suppressive function and the drug efficacy of PARP inhibitors [1–3]. On the other hand, in terms of biochemical properties, BRCA1 has the enzymatic activity of a ubiquitin ligase. We found that BRCA1 forms a RING heterodimer with BARD1 and has a significant E3 ubiquitin ligase activity that is abolished by a patient-derived mutation [4]. Since then, various efforts in this field have been attempted to elucidate the molecular mechanisms, as well as the biological and clinical significance of this activity. This chapter summarizes the evidence on BRCA1 E3 activity, including its role in HR, PARP inhibitor sensitivity, and cancer susceptibility. Because the RING finger domain, which represents only 5% of total BRCA1 protein, contains approximately 60% of pathogenic missense mutations for HBOC [5)], understanding the enzymatic activity of this domain is crucial for the role of BRCA1 in general.

1.2 Biochemical Function of BRCA1 E3 Ligase

1.2.1 Structure and Protein-Protein Interaction of BRCA1

BRCA1 consists of several well-characterized functional domains, including an N-terminal RING finger, exon 11 containing a long disordered region, a coiled-coil domain, and a C-terminal tandem BRCT repeat (Fig. 1.1). BRCA1 forms four distinct complexes with Abraxas (also called ABRA1), FANCJ (also called BACH1 or BRIP1), and CtIP via the C-terminal BRCT domain and PALB2/BRCA2 via the coiled-coil domain, which play essential roles in homologous recombination (HR) repair of DNA double-strand breaks (DSBs) [6–16]. The helicase and nuclease activities of FANCJ and CtIP, respectively, induce the dissociation of double-stranded DNA and single-strand formation at the site of damage [9–13], while PALB2/BRCA2 directs the recombinase RAD51 to this single strand and promotes the formation of DNA-RAD51 filaments required for homology search in sister chromatids [14–16]. Abraxas induces BRCA1 on polyubiquitin chains formed at DNA damage sites via RAP80, which is thought to rather repress and fine-tune HR [17, 18]. In all four of these complexes, BRCA1 forms a RING dimeric core complex with BARD1 [4, 19–21]. Like the zinc-finger motif, the RING finger motif binds to two zinc molecules via four pairs of cysteine or histidine residues that stabilizes the structure [21]; the RING finger of BRCA1 has seven cysteine residues and one histidine residue (Fig. 1.1).

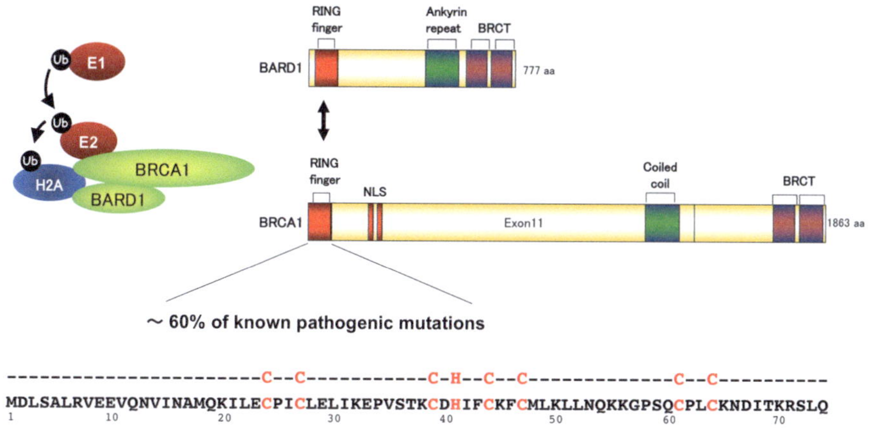

Fig. 1.1 Domain structure of BRCA1 and BARD1. Both BRCA1 and BARD1 have an N-terminal RING finger domain and a C-terminal tandem BRCT domain, which join at the RING finger domain to form a dimer. RING finger is a motif with E3 ubiquitin ligase activity and consists of four-pair of cysteine and histidine residues that binds to two molecules of zinc. Ubiquitin activation and conjugation pathway comprising E1, E2, and BRCA1/BARD1 E3 ligase is shown with a substrate histone H2A

1.2.2 Ubiquitination Catalyzed by BRCA1/BARD1

Covalent ubiquitin conjugation, one of the posttranslational modifications of proteins, regulates various intracellular protein-protein interactions and signal transduction. Signaling by ubiquitin modification depends on the type of the polyubiquitin chains: polyubiquitin chains linked via Lys48 or Lys11 residue of ubiquitin are recognized by the 26S proteasome and signal proteolysis, whereas polyubiquitin chains linked via Lys63 and Lys6 play an important role in the DNA damage response [22–24]. Mono-ubiquitin conjugation is also critical in many cellular mechanisms [25]. The ubiquitin conjugation system consists of three enzymes: a ubiquitin-activating enzyme (E1), a ubiquitin-conjugating enzyme (E2), and a ubiquitin ligase (E3) [26, 27]. Ubiquitin monomers that have been activated by the E1 are transferred to E2. E3 bridges E2-ubiquitin conjugates and its specific substrate and catalyzes the formation of polyubiquitin chains or mono-ubiquitination, onto the substrate via covalent bond (Fig. 1.1). The RING finger is a motif that is responsible for the binding with E2-ubiquitin conjugates [28]. Since our discovery that this motif is required for the E3 activity of ROC1, the catalytic RING finger subunit of the SKP1/CUL1/F-box (SCF) E3 ligase complex [29, 30], hundreds of RING-type E3 ligases have been identified. One such protein, BRCA1, was found to constitute a RING heterodimeric E3 ligase with BARD1 [4, 19–21]. Whereas the RING domain of BRCA1 interacts with E2-ubiquitin conjugates, that of BARD1 does not [21, 31, 32]. BARD1 interacts with BRCA1 on the opposite side of the cleft of the E2-binding site of BRCA1, which is essential for the stability and the E3 ligase activity of BRCA1. BRCA1 alone does not have any E3 ligase activity [4]. The BRCA1/BARD1 catalyzed Lys6-linked polyubiquitin chains, which was identified by mutational and a mass-spectrometric analyses [33–35]. However, the type of polyubiquitin chains catalyzed by BRCA1 is distinct according to E2s and substrates and BRCA1 was found to monoubiquitinate histone H2A and estrogen receptor α (ERα) [32, 36–39].

1.2.3 Substrates of the BRCA1/BARD1 E3 Ligase

Candidate substrates for the BRCA1/BARD1 E3 ligase, including histones, histone chaperone NPM1, C-terminal BRCA1-binding protein CtIP, estrogen receptor α, progesterone receptor-A, the largest subunit of RNA polymerase II RPB1, common subunit of RNA polymerases RPB8, the general transcription factor TFIIE and γ-tubulin, have been previously reported [39–47]. Unfortunately, specific roles in physiological conditions for most of these substrates remain largely unknown. Among them, however, biological significance of H2A ubiquitination by BRCA1/BARD1 has been intensively elucidated.

Mono-ubiquitination of histone H2A by BRCA1/BARD1 was first demonstrated by in vitro reaction using purified H2A protein [48, 49]. In this condition, other histones tested were also ubiquitinated and the reaction was thought to be nonspecific. However, a decade later, when BRCA1/BARD1 was incubated with native chromatin or recombinant nucleosomes reconstituted with histone octamers and DNA, only H2A was ubiquitinated [37]. H2A is ubiquitinated by three crucial E3 ligases at different Lysine residues, leading to distinct biological outcome. Monoubiquitination of H2A at C-terminal Lys118/119 by RING1B/BMI1 of PRC1 polycomb complex mediates transcriptional silencing [50, 51]. Monoubiquitin conjugate at Lys13/15 of H2A produced by RNF168 recruits 53BP1 at DSB sites that promotes nonhomologous end joining (NHEJ) [52, 53]. The monoubiquitination at Lys13/15 of H2A plays another role. When H2A is monoubiquitinated at Lys13/15 by RNF168, another E3 RNF8 further processes the monoubiquitin of this residue into a Lys63-bound polyubiquitin chain [54]. This polyubiquitin chain recruits the BRCA1/Abraxas complex via the ubiquitin-interacting protein RAP80 [6–8]. On the other hand, the residues ubiquitinated by BRCA1/BARD1 is Lys125/127/129, the most C-terminus of H2A [37]. Crystal structure analysis revealed that interaction of BRCA1 and BARD1 with H2A via Arg71 residue of BRCA1 and Trp91 residue of BARD1, respectively, is critical for this reaction [38, 55]. The BRCA1/BARD1 heterodimer is structurally very similar to polycomb RING1B/BMI1 and both monoubiquitinate C-terminal of H2A but slightly different sites: Lys118/119 for RING1B/BMI1 and Lys125/127/129 for BRCA1/BARD1 [37, 38, 55]. Substitution of Lys70 and Arg71 residues of BRCA1 with alanine abolished ubiquitination of H2A mediated by BRCA1/BARD1. This ubiquitination is critical for HR and carcinogenesis as described below.

1.3 Biological Significance of E3 Activity of BRCA1

1.3.1 BRCA1 E3 Ligase Maintains Satellite Heterochromatin

The biological significance of the E3 ligase activity of BRCA1 was first demonstrated in a report that showed that ubiquitination of the histone H2A C-terminus by BRCA1 is essential for heterochromatin-mediated DNA silencing of the satellite region, thereby suppressing oncogenesis [36]. It was shown that ectopic expression of H2A artificially fused with ubiquitin at the C-terminus can rescue the phenotype caused by deletion of BRCA1, indicating that BRCA1 maintains heterochromatin structure via ubiquitylation of histone H2A. Considering that BRCA1 is capable of binding to histone H3 with methylated Lys9 residues (H3K9me) via HP1 bound to BARD1 [56–59], it could be possible that polycomb is responsible for H2A ubiquitination in the H3K27me region [60, 61] and BRCA1/BARD1 for H2A ubiquitination in H3K9me regions such as satellites, contributing to the heterochromatin formation in each of these regions.

1.3.2 BRCA1 E3 Ligase Executes HR

With regard to the significance of the E3 activity of BRCA1 in HR, this activity was shown to remove 53BP1 at DNA damage sites. The most frequently used DSB repair pathways are the aforementioned HR and NHEJ: HR is an error-free repair of DSBs using sister chromatids as templates in the S and G2 phases of the cell cycle, whereas NHEJ is a method of directly joining the blunt ends of DSBs in situations where HR is not available, such as in G1 phase [1–3]. Incidentally, single-strand annealing or PARP1/2-mediated alternative end joining operates as a backup mechanism in situations where none of these are available, e.g., DSBs with clipped, non-blunt ends or one-ended DSBs in BRCA1/2 deletions [62]. In general, HR and NHEJ inhibit each other, with BRCA1/2 acting as the guardian of HR, whereas 53BP1 is the guardian of NHEJ, i.e., 53BP1 induces downstream repair factors required for NHEJ [63–72] (Fig. 1.2). During the repair process of DSBs, BRCA1 localizes to the center of damage and 53BP1 surrounds it, whereas in BRCA1-deficient cells, 53BP1 accumulates at the central site of damage [73–75]. This means that one of the important roles of BRCA1 is to move 53BP1 away from the site of injury. Notably, the E3 activity of BRCA1 is responsible for this process, which is most important in the early stages of homologous recombination repair. The mechanism is via monoubiquitination of the histone H2A C-terminus, Lys127/128/129, by BRCA1, which recruits SMARCAD1, an ATP-dependent motor protein that executes chromatin remodeling [76, 77]. SMARCAD1 moves the entire histone octamer, with which 53BP1 interacts via monoubiquitination of Lys15 of H2A, from the center to the periphery of the DNA damage region (Fig. 1.2). The resulting naked double-stranded DNA is unwound by helicases, and

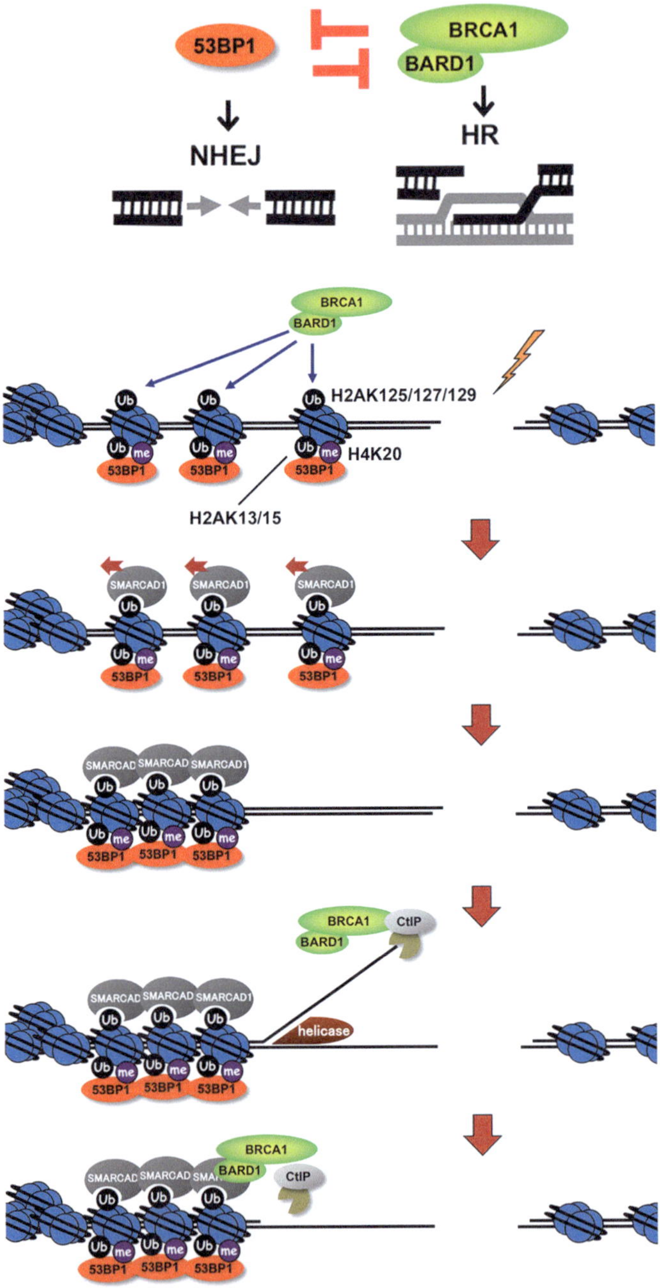

Fig. 1.2 HR mediated by BRCA1 E3 activity. The two major DSB repair pathways, NHEJ and HR, are promoted by 53BP1 and BRCA1, respectively, and mutually repress each other; BRCA1 ubiquitinates histone H2A that recruits a chromatin remodeler SMARCAD1 to move the entire 53BP1-bound histone octamer away from the site of DNA damage. This inhibits NHEJ, and BRCA1 subsequently assists CtIP to create single-stranded DNA overhang, which is then bound by RAD51 for homologous recombination repair

BRCA1-induced CtIP, in collaboration with endonuclease activity of MRE11, degrades 5′-terminated DNA strand, forming a single-stranded DNA overhang, which slides into the sister chromatid via RAD51, thus undergoing homologous recombination [12, 13, 62, 78, 79].

1.4 Clinical Significance of E3 Activity of BRCA1

1.4.1 E3 Activity Prevents HBOC Carcinogenesis

In our first report of E3 activity in BRCA1, we showed that a Cys61Gly mutation resulting from hereditary breast cancer abolished E3 activity in BRCA1 [4]. However, the phenotype could not be described as a purely E3 activity-dead phenotype, as it inhibits binding to BARD1 that disrupts various functions of BRCA1, including protein stability. In contrast, in collaboration with Dr. Rachel Klevit's crystallography, we found that the Ile26Ala mutation inhibited the E3 activity of BRCA1 while maintaining its binding to BARD1 [21] (Fig. 1.3, E3). The residue Ile26 was essential for BRCA1 to bind UbcH5c, the E2 most frequently used in ubiquitin studies [31)]. Subsequently, a great deal of work has been done with this Ile26Ala mutation to date. One of the most important reports concerns carcinogenesis in mice. Dr. Thomas Ludwig and his group, an authority on mouse BRCA carcinogenesis models, have used a conditional mammary gland-specific knock-in mouse model in which *BRCA1* mutations are introduced together with *TP53* mutations, and found that BRCT mutations in *BRCA1* develop breast carcinogenesis, whereas Ile26Ala knock-in mice do not, and their embryonic fibroblasts (MEFs) have HR repair capacity comparable to wild-type for the DNA cross-linker mitomycin C [80]. However, there is a profound contradiction between this finding and the fact that mutations in the BRCA1 RING finger domain that maintain interaction with BRAD1 but eliminate E3 activity are actually classified as pathogenic missense mutations [5, 21, 81–85] (Fig. 1.3, E3). One possibility is that different species may have different severity for phenotypes, i.e., breast cancer in humans but not in mice. For example, unlike humans, a deletion of one allele of BRCA1 does not cause cancer in mice. Previous models of carcinogenesis have been deletion of exon 11 of *BRCA1* crossed with deletion of p53, or organ-specific knockout or mutations of both alleles [86]. In addition to that, it has been shown that the Ile26Ala mutation is not a completely dead mutation but sufficiently active depending on the type of partner, E2 [87]. Furthermore, the Ile26Ala/Leu63Ala/Lys65Ala triple mutant, which can completely abolish the activity toward H2A in the nucleosome while maintaining binding to BARD1, has been shown to inhibit HR and markedly increase cell sensitivity to DNA-damaging agents including mitomycin C [85].

In addition to mutations in the E2-binding site, mutations in the H2A-binding site of BRCA1 and BARD1 can also inhibit H2A ubiquitination by BRCA1; residue

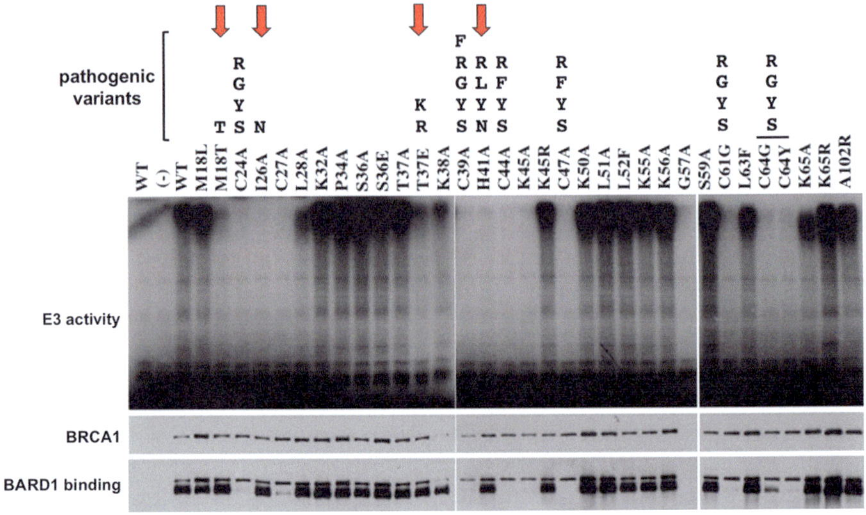

Fig. 1.3 Effect of BRCA1 mutations in the RING finger domain on BARD1 binding and E3 activity. Cell lysates from 293 T cells expressing either wild-type or mutant myc-BRCA1(1–772) with or without (lane 1) HA-BARD1 were immunoprecipitated with anti-Myc antibody. The precipitates were examined for a substrate-independent E3 ligase assay with E2 UbcH5c, or immunoblotted with BRCA1 or BARD1. Pathogenic variants indicated in ClinVar database are shown at the top. Red arrows indicate mutants that inhibit or likely inhibit E3 ligase activity but retain the BARD1 binding. Different similar datasets within this series of experiments have been published previously in reference [21]

Lys71 of BRCA1 is a binding site for H2A and mutations in this site do not inhibit BRCA1 E3 activity but inhibit activity against H2A [38, 55]. Importantly, the variants at this site, R71G, R71M, and R71L, are pathogenic mutations. Furthermore, hereditary BARD1 missense mutations in the RING finger motif found in familial breast cancer that affect zinc binding, C53W, C71Y, and C83R, retained the ability to form a heterodimeric complex with BRCA1 to make active ubiquitin ligase, but binding to nucleosomes and activity to ubiquitinate histone H2A was defective [88]. These lines of evidence suggest that the E3 activity of BRCA1, particularly its ability to ubiquitinate histone H2A, is crucial in preventing cancer.

Several functional assessment methods have now been devised in predicting cancer development in VUS, including HR capacity and PARP inhibitor sensitivity [81–84, 89]. Given that HR failure is the most critical factor in cancer development, it is direct to analyze HR capacity, but assessment is not always straightforward. Traditionally, the evaluation of HR capacity using a reporter gene that fluoresces when GFP with cleaved coding regions is repaired by recombination has been widely used, but this method uses an exogenous DNA reporter and does not take into account chromosomal conditions such as heterochromatin, so it may not fully reflect actual in vivo HR capacity. With this in mind, a method of directly cleaving genomic DNA in cells with CRISPR/Cas9 has been devised and is expected to be useful [84]. However, each functional analysis has its advantages and disadvantages, and E3 activity, the only enzymatic activity of BRCA1, is certainly an important tool in the prediction of VUS carcinogenesis.

1.4.2 E3 Activity Affects PARP Inhibitor Sensitivity

Apart from its effect on carcinogenesis, another clinically important phenotype of BRCA1 dysfunction is PARP inhibitor hypersensitivity. Although an artificial variant, the complete E3-dead mutant of BRCA1, Ile26Ala/Leu63Ala/Lys65Ala, showed a markedly increased sensitivity to PARP inhibitor olaparib [85]. Moderate enhanced sensitivity to olaparib has also been reported with Ile26Ala alone [76, 84, 85]. Furthermore, mutations in BARD1 that abolish BRCA1 E3 activity also suppress HR and increase sensitivity to olaparib [76, 85]. These lines of evidence suggest that suppression of BRCA1 E3 activity causes PARP inhibitor susceptibility, and in addition to its clinical importance as a predictive marker of susceptibility, agents that control this activity may also be useful as a therapeutic strategy in the future.

Perspectives

As vast amounts of clinical data accumulate, it is likely that variants once thought to be VUS would be shown to be pathogenic or nonpathogenic. However, it is also true that new VUS will be detected along the way. Functional analysis is still important to predict carcinogenesis of these VUS without sufficient support from clinical data, and the evaluation of E3 activity will continue to be important. It is essential to provide patients with more appropriate treatment based on sufficient clinical data and in vitro functional analyses.

References

1. Silver DP, Livingston DM. Mechanisms of BRCA1 tumor suppression. Cancer Discov. 2012;2(8):679–84.
2. Ciccia A, Elledge SJ. The DNA damage response: making it safe to play with knives. Mol Cell. 2010;40(2):179–204.
3. Tarsounas M, Sung P. The antitumorigenic roles of BRCA1-BARD1 in DNA repair and replication. Nat Rev Mol Cell Biol. 2020;21(5):284–99.
4. Hashizume R, Fukuda M, Maeda I, et al. The RING heterodimer BRCA1-BARD1 is a ubiquitin ligase inactivated by a breast cancer-derived mutation. J Biol Chem. 2001;276:14537–40.
5. Starita LM, Young DL, Islam M, Kitzman JO, Gullingsrud J, Hause RJ, Fowler DM, Parvin JD, Shendure J, Fields S. Massively parallel functional analysis of BRCA1 RING domain variants. Genetics. 2015;200:413–22.
6. Wang B, Matsuoka S, Ballif BA, et al. Abraxas and RAP80 form a BRCA1 protein complex required for the DNA damage response. Science. 2007;316:1194–8.
7. Sobhian B, Shao G, Lilli DR, et al. RAP80 targets BRCA1 to specific ubiquitin structures at DNA damage sites. Science. 2007;316:1198–202.

8. Kim H, Chen J, Yu X. Ubiquitin-binding protein RAP80 mediates BRCA1-dependent DNA damage response. Science. 2007;316:1202–5.
9. Cantor SB, Bell DW, Ganesan S, et al. BACH1, a novel helicase-like protein, interacts directly with BRCA1 and contributes to its DNA repair function. Cell. 2001;105:149–60.
10. Litman R, Peng M, Jin Z, et al. BACH1 is critical for homologous recombination and appears to be the Fanconi anemia gene product FANCJ. Cancer Cell. 2005;8:255–65.
11. Yu X, Wu LC, Bowcock AM, et al. The C-terminal (BRCT) domains of BRCA1 interact in vivo with CtIP, a protein implicated in the CtBP pathway of transcriptional repression. J Biol Chem. 1998;273:25388–92.
12. Sartori AA, Lukas C, Coates J, et al. Human CtIP promotes DNA end resection. Nature. 2007;450:509–14.
13. Yun MH, Hiom K. CtIP-BRCA1 modulates the choice of DNA double-strand-break repair pathway throughout the cell cycle. Nature. 2009;459:460–3.
14. Zhang F, Ma J, Wu J, et al. PALB2 links BRCA1 and BRCA2 in the DNA-damage response. Curr Biol. 2009;19:524–9.
15. Sy SMH, Huen MSY, Chen J. PALB2 is an integral component of the BRCA complex required for homologous recombination repair. Proc Natl Acad Sci USA. 2009;106:7155–60.
16. Oliver AW, Swift S, Lord CJ. Structural basis for recruitment of BRCA2 by PALB2. EMBO Rep. 2009;10:990–6.
17. Hu Y, Scully R, Sobhian B, et al. RAP80-directed tuning of BRCA1 homologous recombination function at ionizing radiation-induced nuclear foci. Genes Dev. 2011;25:685–700.
18. Coleman KA, Greenberg RA. The BRCA1-RAP80 complex regulates DNA repair mechanism utilization by restricting end resection. J Biol Chem. 2011;286:13669–80.
19. Wu LC, Wang ZW, Tsan JT, et al. Identification of a RING protein that can interact in vivo with the BRCA1 gene product. Nat Genet. 1996;14:430–40.
20. Meza JE, Brzovic PS, King MC, Klevit RE. Mapping the functional domains of BRCA1. Interaction of the ring finger domains of BRCA1 and BARD1. J Biol Chem. 1999;274(9):5659–65.
21. Brzovic PS, Keeffe JR, Nishikawa H, et al. Binding and recognition in the assembly of an active BRCA1/BARD1 ubiquitin-ligase complex. Proc Natl Acad Sci USA. 2003;100:646–5651.
22. Pickart CM. Back to the future with ubiquitin. Cell. 2004;116:181–90.
23. Mukhopadhyay D, Riezman H. Proteasome-independent functions of ubiquitin in endocytosis and signaling. Science. 2007;315(5809):201–5.
24. Ohta T, Fukuda M. Ubiquitin and breast cancer. Oncogene. 2004;23(11):2079–88.
25. Hicke L. Protein regulation by monoubiquitin. Nat Rev Mol Cell Biol. 2001;2(3):195–201.
26. Hershko A, Ciechanover A. The ubiquitin system. Annu Rev Biochem. 1998;67:425–79.
27. Pickart CM, Eddins MJ. Ubiquitin: structures, functions, mechanisms. Biochim Biophys Acta. 2004;1695(1–3):55–72.
28. Lorick KL, Jensen JP, Fang S, Ong AM, Hatakeyama S, Weissman AM. RING fingers mediate ubiquitin-conjugating enzyme (E2)-dependent ubiquitination. Proc Natl Acad Sci USA. 1999;96(20):11364–9.
29. Ohta T, Michel JJ, Schottelius AJ, Xiong Y. ROC1, a homolog of APC11, represents a family of cullin partners with an associated ubiquitin ligase activity. Mol Cell. 1999;3(4):535–41.
30. Furukawa M, Ohta T, Xiong Y. Activation of UBC5 ubiquitin-conjugating enzyme by the RING finger of ROC1 and assembly of active ubiquitin ligases by all cullins. J Biol Chem. 2002;277(18):15758–65.
31. Brzovic PS, Lissounov A, Christensen DE, Hoyt DW, Klevit RE. A UbcH5/ubiquitin noncovalent complex is required for processive BRCA1-directed ubiquitination. Mol Cell. 2006;21(6):873–80.
32. Christensen DEB, PS, Klevit RE. E2-BRCA1 RING interactions dictate synthesis of mono- or specific polyubiquitin chain linkages. Nat Struct Mol Biol. 2007;14(10):941–8.

33. Wu-Baer F, Lagrazon K, Yuan W, Baer R. The BRCA1/BARD1 heterodimer assembles polyubiquitin chains through an unconventional linkage involving lysine residue K6 of ubiquitin. J Biol Chem. 2003;278(37):34743–6.
34. Nishikawa H, Ooka S, Sato K, Arima K, Okamoto J, Klevit RE, Fukuda M, Ohta T. Mass spectrometric and mutational analyses reveal Lys-6-linked polyubiquitin chains catalyzed by BRCA1-BARD1 ubiquitin ligase. J Biol Chem. 2004;279(6):3916–24.
35. Morris JR, Solomon E. BRCA1: BARD1 induces the formation of conjugated ubiquitin structures, dependent on K6 of ubiquitin, in cells during DNA replication and repair. Hum Mol Genet. 2004;13(8):807–17.
36. Zhu Q, Pao GM, Huynh AM, Suh H, Tonnu N, Nederlof PM, Gage FH, Verma IM. BRCA1 tumour suppression occurs via heterochromatin-mediated silencing. Nature. 2011;477:179–84.
37. Kalb R, Mallery DL, Larkin C, Huang JTJ, Hiom K. BRCA1 is a histone-H2A-specific ubiquitin ligase. Cell Rep. 2014;8:999–1005.
38. Witus SR, Burrell AL, Farrell DP, Kang J, Wang M, Hansen JM, Pravat A, Tuttle LM, Stewart MD, Brzovic PS, Chatterjee C, Zhao W, DiMaio F, Kollman JM, Klevit RE. BRCA1/BARD1 site-specific ubiquitylation of nucleosomal H2A is directed by BARD1. Nat Struct Mol Biol. 2021;28(3):268–77.
39. Eakin CM, Maccoss MJ, Finney GL, Klevit RE. Estrogen receptor alpha is a putative substrate for the BRCA1 ubiquitin ligase. Proc Natl Acad Sci USA. 2007;104(14):5794–9.
40. Sato K, Hayami R, Wu W, Nishikawa T, Nishikawa H, Okuda Y, Ogata H, Fukuda M, Ohta T. Nucleophosmin/B23 is a candidate substrate for the BRCA1-BARD1 ubiquitin ligase. J Biol Chem. 2004;279(30):30919–22.
41. Yu X, Fu S, Lai M, Baer R, Chen J. BRCA1 ubiquitinates its phosphorylation-dependent binding partner CtIP. Genes Dev. 2006;20(13):1721–6.
42. Poole AJ, Li Y, Kim Y, Lin SC, Lee WH, Lee EY. Prevention of Brca1-mediated mammary tumorigenesis in mice by a progesterone antagonist. Science. 2006;314:1467–70.
43. Kleiman FE, Wu-Baer F, Fonseca D, Kaneko S, Baer R, Manley JL. BRCA1/BARD1 inhibition of mRNA 30 processing involves targeted degradation of RNA polymerase II. Genes Dev. 2005;19:1227–37.
44. Starita LM, Horwitz AA, Keogh MC, Ishioka C, Parvin JD, Chiba N. BRCA1/BARD1 ubiquitinate phosphorylated RNA polymerase II. J Biol Chem. 2005;280:24498–505.
45. Wu W, Nishikawa H, Hayami R, Sato K, Honda A, Aratani S, Nakajima T, Fukuda M, Ohta T. BRCA1 ubiquitinates RPB8 in response to DNA damage. Cancer Res. 2007;67:951–8.
46. Horwitz AA, Affar el B, Heine GF, Shi Y, Parvin JD. A mechanism for transcriptional repression dependent on the BRCA1 E3 ubiquitin ligase. Proc Natl Acad Sci USA. 2007;104:6614–9.
47. Starita LM, Machida Y, Sankaran S, Elias JE, Griffin K, Schlegel BP, Gygi SP, Parvin JD. BRCA1-dependent ubiquitination of gamma-tubulin regulates centrosome number. Mol Cell Biol. 2004;24:8457–66.
48. Chen A, Kleiman FE, Manley JL, Ouchi T, Pan ZQ. Autoubiquitination of the BRCA1/BARD1 RING ubiquitin ligase. J Biol Chem. 2002;277(24):22085–92.
49. Mallery DL, Vandenberg CJ, Hiom K. Activation of the E3 ligase function of the BRCA1/BARD1 complex by polyubiquitin chains. EMBO J. 2002;21(24):6755–62.
50. Wang H, Wang L, Erdjument-Bromage H, Mi V, Tempst P, Jones RS, Zhang Y. Role of histone H2A ubiquitination in Polycomb silencing. Nature. 2004;431(7010):873–8.
51. Simon JA, Kingston RE. Occupying chromatin: polycomb mechanisms for getting to genomic targets, stopping transcriptional traffic, and staying put. Mol Cell. 2013;49:808–24.
52. Fradet-Turcotte A, Canny MD, Escribano-Díaz C, Orthwein A, Leung CC, Huang H, Landry MC, Kitevski-LeBlanc J, Noordermeer SM, Sicheri F, Durocher D. 53BP1 is a reader of the DNA-damage-induced H2A Lys 15 ubiquitin mark. Nature. 2013;499:50–4.
53. Wilson MD, Benlekbir S, Fradet-Turcotte A, Sherker A, Julien JP, McEwan A, Noordermeer SM, Sicheri F, Rubinstein JL, Durocher D. The structural basis of modified nucleosome recognition by 53BP1. Nature. 2016;536:100–3.

54. Mattiroli F, Vissers JHA, van Dijk WJ, Ikpa P, Citterio E, Vermeulen W, Marteijn JA, Sixma TK. RNF168 ubiquitinates K13-15 on H2A/H2AX to drive DNA damage signaling. Cell. 2012;150(6):1182–95.
55. McGinty RK, Henrici RC, Tan S. Crystal structure of the PRC1 ubiquitylation module bound to the nucleosome. Nature. 2014;514(7524):591–6.
56. Wu W, Nishikawa H, Fukuda T, Vittal V, Asano M, Miyoshi Y, Klevit RE, Ohta T. Interaction of BARD1 and HP1 is required for BRCA1 retention at sites of DNA damage. Cancer Res. 2015;75(7):1311–21.
57. Wu W, Togashi Y, Johmura Y, Miyoshi Y, Nobuoka S, Nakanishi M, Ohta T. HP1 regulates the localization of FANCJ at sites of DNA double-strand breaks. Cancer Sci. 2016;107(10):1406–15.
58. Fukuda T, Wu W, Okada M, Maeda I, Kojima Y, Hayami R, Miyoshi Y, Tsugawa K, Ohta T. Class I histone deacetylase inhibitors inhibit the retention of BRCA1 and 53BP1 at the site of DNA damage. Cancer Sci. 2015;106(8):1050–6.
59. Billing D, Horiguchi M, Wu-Baer F, Taglialatela A, Leuzzi G, Nanez SA, Jiang W, Zha S, Szabolcs M, Lin CS, Ciccia A, Baer R. The BRCT domains of the BRCA1 and BARD1 tumor suppressors differentially regulate homology-directed repair and stalled fork protection. Mol Cell. 2018;72(1):127–39.
60. Cao R, Wang L, Wang H, Xia L, Erdjument-Bromage H, Tempst P, Jones RS, Zhang Y. Role of histone H3 lysine 27 methylation in Polycomb-group silencing. Science. 2002;298(5595):1039–43.
61. Margueron R, Reinberg D. The Polycomb complex PRC2 and its mark in life. Natur. 2011;469(7330):343–9.
62. Ceccaldi R, Rondinelli B, D'Andrea AD. Repair pathway choices and consequences at the double-Strand break. Trends Cell Biol. 2016;26(1):52–64.
63. Bunting SF, Callen E, Wong N, et al. 53BP1 inhibits homologous recombination in Brca1-deficient cells by blocking resection of DNA breaks. Cell. 2010;141:243–54.
64. Cao L, Xu X, Bunting SF, et al. A selective requirement for 53BP1 in the biological response to genomic instability induced by Brca1 deficiency. Mol Cell. 2009;35:534–41.
65. Bouwman P, Aly A, Escandell JM, et al. 53BP1 loss rescues BRCA1 deficiency and is associated with triple-negative and BRCA-mutated breast cancers. Nat Struct Mol Biol. 2010;17:688–95.
66. Escribano-Diaz C, Orthwein A, Fradet-Turcotte A, et al. A cell cycle-dependent regulatory circuit composed of 53BP1-RIF1 and BRCA1-CtIP controls DNA repair pathway choice. Mol Cell. 2013;49:872–83.
67. Chapman JP, Barral P, Vannier JB, et al. RIF1 is essential for 53BP1-dependent nonhomologous end joining and suppression of DNA double-strand break resection. Mol Cell. 2013;49:858–71.
68. Zimmermann M, Lottersberger F, Buonomo SB, et al. 53BP1 regulates DSB repair using Rif1 to control 5′ end resection. Science. 2013;339:700–4.
69. Xu G, Chapman JR, Brandsma I. REV7 counteracts DNA double-strand break resection and affects PARP inhibition. Nature. 2015;521:541–4.
70. Noordermeer SM, Adam S, Setiaputra D, et al. The shieldin complex mediates 53BP1-dependent DNA repair. Nature. 2018;560:117–21.
71. Ghezraoui H, Oliveira C, Becker JR, et al. 53BP1 cooperation with the REV7-shieldin complex underpins DNA structure-specific NHEJ. Nature. 2018;560:122–7.
72. Mirman Z, Lottersberger F, Takai H, et al. 53BP1–RIF1–shieldin counteracts DSB resection through CST- and Polα-dependent fill-in. Nature. 2018;560:112–6.
73. Kakarougkas A, Ismail A, Katsuki Y, Freire R, Shibata A, Jeggo PA. Co-operation of BRCA1 and POH1 relieves the barriers posed by 53BP1 and RAP80 to resection. Nucleic Acids Res. 2013;41(22):10298–311.

74. Kakarougkas A, Ismail A, Klement K, Goodarzi AA, Conrad S, Freire R, Shibata A, Lobrich M, Jeggo PA. Opposing roles for 53BP1 during homologous recombination. Nucleic Acids Res. 2013;41(21):9719–31.
75. Alagoz M, Katsuki Y, Ogiwara H, Ogi T, Shibata A, Kakarougkas A, Jeggo P. SETDB1, HP1 and SUV39 promote repositioning of 53BP1 to extend resection during homologous recombination in G2 cells. Nucleic Acids Res. 2015;43(16):7931–44.
76. Densham RM, Garvin AJ, Stone HR, Strachan J, Baldock RA, Daza-Martin M, Fletcher A, Blair-Reid S, Beesley J, Pearl LH JB, Neely R, Keep NH, Watts FZ, Morris JR. Human BRCA1-BARD1 ubiquitin ligase activity counteracts chromatin barriers to DNA resection. Nat Struct Mol Biol. 2016;23(7):647–55.
77. Densham RM, Morris JR. The BRCA1 ubiquitin ligase function sets a new trend for remodelling in DNA repair. Nucleus. 2017;8(2):116–25.
78. Pellegrini L, Yu DS, Lo T, et al. Insights into DNA recombination from the structure of a RAD51-BRCA2 complex. Nature. 2002;420:287–93.
79. Zhao W, Steinfeld JB, Liang F, Chen X, Maranon DG, Ma Jian C, Kwon Y, Rao T, Wang W, Sheng C, et al. BRCA1-BARD1 promotes. RAD51-mediated homologous DNA pairing. Nature. 2017;550:360–5.
80. Shakya R, Reid LJ, Reczek CR, Cole F, Egli D, Lin CS, deRooij DG, Hirsch S, Ravi K, Hicks JB, Szabolcs M, Jasin M, Baer R, Ludwig T. BRCA1 tumor suppression depends on BRCT phosphoprotein binding, but not its E3 ligase activity. Science. 2011;334:525–8.
81. Morris JR, Pangon L, Boutell C, Katagiri T, Keep NH, Solomon E. Genetic analysis of BRCA1 ubiquitin ligase activity and its relationship to breast cancer susceptibility. Hum Mol Genet. 2006;15:599–606.
82. Ransburgh DJR, Chiba N, Ishioka C, Toland AE, Parvin JD. Identification of breast tumor mutations in BRCA1 that abolish its function in homologous DNA recombination. Cancer Res. 2010;70(3):988–95.
83. Towler WI, Zhang J, Ransburgh DJR, Toland AE, Ishioka C, Chiba N, Parvin JD. Analysis of BRCA1 variants in double-strand break repair by homologous recombination and single-strand annealing. Hum Mutat. 2013;34(3):439–45.
84. Yoshino Y, Endo S, Chen Z, Qi H, Watanabe G, Chiba N. Evaluation of site-specific homologous recombination activity of BRCA1 by direct quantitation of gene editing efficiency. Sci Rep. 2019;9(1):1644.
85. Wang M, Li W, Tomimatsu N, Yu CH, Ji JH, Alejo S, Witus SR, Alimbetov D, Fitzgerald O, Wu B, Wang Q, Huang Y, Gan Y, Dong F, Kwon Y, Sareddy GR, Curiel TJ, Habib AA, Hromas R, Dos Santos PC, Yao T, Ivanov DN, Brzovic PS, Burma S, Klevit RE, Zhao W. Crucial roles of the BRCA1-BARD1 E3 ubiquitin ligase activity in homology-directed DNA repair. Mol Cell. 2023;83(20):3679–91.
86. Dine J, Deng CX. Mouse models of BRCA1 and their application to breast cancer research. Cancer Metastasis Rev. 2013;32(1–2):25–37.
87. Stewart MD, Duncan ED, Coronado E, DaRosa PA, Pruneda JN, Brzovic PS, Klevit RE. Tuning BRCA1 and BARD1 activity to investigate RING ubiquitin ligase mechanisms. Protein Sci. 2017;26(3):475–83.
88. Stewart MD, Zeli E, Dhall A, Walsh T, Upadhyay E, Corn JE, Chatterjee C, King MC, Klevit RE. BARD1 is necessary for ubiquitylation of nucleosomal histone H2A and for transcriptional regulation of estrogen metabolism genes. Proc Natl Acad Sci USA. 2018;115(6):1316–21.
89. Ikegami M, Kohsaka S, Ueno T, Momozawa Y, Inoue S, Tamura K, Shimomura A, Hosoya N, Kobayashi H, Tanaka S, Mano H. High-throughput functional evaluation of BRCA2 variants of unknown significance. Nat Commun. 2020;11(1):2573.

Chapter 2
Mechanisms Underlying the Resistance to Platinum and PARP Inhibitors in *BRCA1/2*-Mutated Tumors

Toshiyasu Taniguchi

Abstract Platinum agents have been used in the treatment of ovarian cancer, and recently, PARP inhibitors have also been increasingly utilized, especially in cases with mutations in *BRCA1* or *BRCA2*, or those with homologous recombination deficiencies. Acquired resistance to platinum and PARP inhibitors has become a clinically important issue. Various mechanisms of resistance have been proposed, among which "functional restoration through secondary mutations in *BRCA1* or *BRCA2* (reversion mutation)" holds clinical importance. This chapter provides an overview of recent insights into the molecular mechanisms of PARP inhibitor resistance, with a focus on secondary mutations in *BRCA1* or *BRCA2*.

2.1 Introduction

Platinum agents, such as carboplatin, cisplatin, and oxaliplatin, have been widely used in the treatment of various types of malignant tumors, including ovarian cancer. Recently, poly (ADP-ribose) polymerase (PARP) inhibitors have also been employed in the treatment of ovarian cancer, breast cancer, pancreatic cancer, and castration-resistant prostate cancer [1].

In 2009, high success rates in the phase 1 clinical trials of a PARP inhibitor, olaparib (Lynparza), were reported in various *BRCA*-mutation-related tumors [2]. Subsequently, numerous reports demonstrating the effectiveness of PARP inhibitors in ovarian cancer [3–7], breast cancer [8–11], pancreatic cancer [12], and prostate cancer [13–16] have been published, allowing PARP inhibitors to be used in actual

T. Taniguchi (✉)
Department of Molecular Life Science, Tokai University School of Medicine, Isehara, Kanagawa, Japan
e-mail: ttanigu-tky@umin.ac.jp

T. Ohta et al. (eds.), *Practical Guide to Hereditary Breast and Ovarian Cancer III*, https://doi.org/10.1007/978-981-96-6779-6_2

clinical practice. However, the acquisition of resistance to platinum and PARP inhibitors has become a significant clinical problem [1, 17].

Individuals carrying pathogenic variants (mutations) in one allele of *BRCA1* or *BRCA2* exhibit hereditary breast and ovarian cancer syndrome (HBOC), which is inherited in an autosomal dominant manner. HBOC predisposes individuals to a higher risk of developing breast cancer, ovarian cancer, pancreatic cancer, prostate cancer, as well as cancers of other organs such as the esophagus, stomach, and bile ducts [18]. On the other hand, individuals carrying pathogenic variants in both alleles of *BRCA1* or *BRCA2*, inherited from both paternal and maternal sides, develop Fanconi anemia (FA), an autosomal recessive disorder [19, 20]. The responsible gene for FA-S complementation group of FA is *BRCA1*, and that for FA-D1 complementation group is *BRCA2*; hence *BRCA1* is also known as *FANCS* and *BRCA2* as *FANCD1*.

Both BRCA1 and BRCA2 are involved in DNA repair, especially homologous recombination repair [21, 22], replication fork protection [23, 24], and replication gap suppression (ssDNA gap suppression) [25–30].

Among them, homologous recombination repair is reported to have the pivotal function that affects tumorigenesis and therapy response [31, 32]. Experiments with separation-of-function mutants of *BRCA2* suggest that BRCA2 promotes therapeutic resistance primarily through homologous recombination, not through replication fork protection or ssDNA gap suppression [31–33].

DNA repair is crucial for both the development and treatment of cancer. DNA damaged by various internal and external factors is repaired by various DNA repair mechanisms. However, when DNA repair is defective, cells may undergo cell death due to incomplete repair, or mutations may accumulate, promoting carcinogenesis. Conversely, DNA repair abnormalities can be exploited as weaknesses in cancer cells for treatment. For instance, cancer cells with abnormalities in homologous recombination repair exhibit high sensitivity to PARP inhibitors [1] and DNA interstrand cross-linking agents, such as platinum compounds [34].

High sensitivity to platinum agents of cancer cells with dysfunctional BRCA1 or BRCA2 can be partly explained by the involvement of BRCA1 or BRCA2 in repairing interstrand DNA crosslinks induced by platinum agents [34]. Recently, a model proposing that excessive single-strand DNA (ssDNA) gaps formed during DNA replication in BRCA1 or BRCA2-deficient cells contribute to platinum sensitivity has also been proposed [28].

Synthetic lethality refers to the concept where combinations of mutations that are not lethal individually become lethal when combined [35, 36]. Dysfunctional homologous recombination combined with PARP inhibition represents a synthetic lethal combination. Therefore, tumors with abnormalities in homologous recombination, such as those with *BRCA1* or *BRCA2* mutations, exhibit sensitivity to PARP inhibitors [37, 38]. Initially, it was interpreted that inhibition of single-strand break repair by PARP inhibition leads to conversion of single-strand breaks to double-strand breaks during DNA replication, which are then repaired by homologous recombination requiring functional BRCA1 or BRCA2, resulting in lethality in BRCA1/2 deficiency. Subsequently, a model proposing that PARP inhibitors trap

PARP itself on DNA upon inhibiting PARP auto-ADP-ribosylation, leading to replication stress, which cells cannot cope with in the absence of functional BRCA1 or BRCA2, was suggested [39, 40]. This model is called the "PARP trapping model" and is now widely accepted [41].

Even tumors without germline mutations in *BRCA1* or *BRCA2* may exhibit a BRCA1- or BRCA2-deficient-like state, termed "BRCAness" [42]. Conditions that can induce BRCAness include germline and/or somatic mutations in genes involved in homologous recombination (*PALB2*, Fanconi anemia genes, RAD51 paralogs (*RAD51B*, *RAD51C*, *RAD51D*), *ATM*, *ATR*, *CDK12*, *CHK1*, *CHK2*, *NBN*, *BRIP1*, *MRE11A*, *BLM*, etc.), and inactivation of *BRCA1* by promoter methylation of *BRCA1* gene [43, 44]. Approximately half of ovarian cancers exhibit homologous recombination deficiency (BRCAness), and PARP inhibitors are expected to be effective in these cases [45]. Additionally, PARP inhibitors may also be effective in ovarian cancers without obvious homologous recombination deficiency [46, 47]. Therefore, it cannot be simply concluded that "BRCA1 or BRCA2 dysfunction equals effectiveness of PARP inhibitors." However, tumors with BRCA1 or BRCA2 deficiency serve as useful models for studying resistance mechanisms, and in this chapter, we focus on PARP inhibitor resistance mechanisms in BRCA1- or BRCA2-deficient tumors (Fig. 2.1). As expected from the usefulness of clinical platinum sensitivity as a marker to predict response to PARP inhibitors [3], mechanisms of platinum resistance and PARP inhibitor resistance share some commonalities. Various mechanisms of PARP inhibitor resistance have been proposed, including functional restoration of BRCA1/BRCA2 by *BRCA1/BRCA2* reversion mutations, BRCA1/2 partial functional restoration through utilization of *BRCA1/2* mutant alleles, elevated RAD51 protein levels in BRCA2-deficient cancer cells, BRCA1 expression restoration in *BRCA1*-methylated tumors, deficiency of 53BP1-related factors in BRCA1-deficient tumors, restoration of replication fork protection, ssDNA gap suppression, increased extracellular drug efflux via p-glycoprotein upregulation, reduced PARP1/2 trapping (*PARP1* mutations, loss of PARG, overexpression of ALC1, etc.), and others [1, 17, 48].

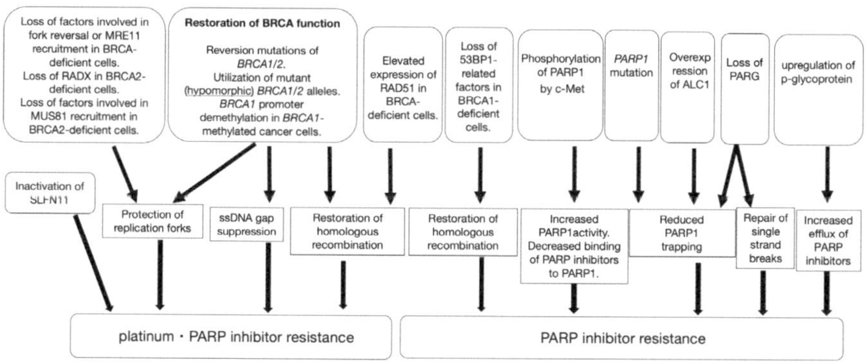

Fig. 2.1 Major mechanisms of platinum/PARP inhibitor resistance in BRCA1/2-deficient tumors (see text for details)

2.2 Functional Restoration of BRCA1/2 by Secondary Mutations (Reversion Mutations) in *BRCA1* and *BRCA2*

If the mechanism of drug sensitivity involves DNA repair abnormalities, it is reasonable to speculate that restoration of DNA repair will be crucial as a mechanism of drug resistance acquisition. In particular, the phenomenon of reversion mutations in *BRCA1/BRCA2* itself (secondary mutations causing functional recovery) is now well known as a common mechanism of resistance acquisition to platinum drugs and PARP inhibitors in *BRCA1/2*-mutated tumors [49].

In 2008, Ashworth's group and our group reported that functional restoration of BRCA1 and BRCA2 proteins by secondary mutations in *BRCA1* and *BRCA2* themselves (reversion mutations) is a common mechanism for acquiring resistance to platinum and PARP inhibitors in *BRCA1*-mutated and *BRCA2*-mutated tumors [50–53]. For example, if the original *BRCA* mutation causes a frameshift, a secondary mutation that cancels out this frameshift can occur, resulting in the tumor expressing a BRCA protein with nearly normal function (Fig. 2.2). There are various types of *BRCA1/2* reversion mutations, including second-site deletions/insertions, which cancel the frameshift caused by the original mutations, in-frame deletions surrounding the original mutation site, and back mutations that completely revert to the wild type [54].

While the mechanism of reversion mutation is not fully understood, microhomology-mediated end joining (MMEJ) may play a major role in occurrence of some of the reversion deletions/insertion mutations, since sometimes short sequences of microhomology at the ends of the site of reversion mutations are observed [54–56]. MMEJ acts as one of the backups to repair DNA double-strand breaks when HR is not functioning. DNA polymerase θ (polθ), encoded by the *POLQ* gene, is a one of the key players of MMEJ [57], and MMEJ is later termed polymerase theta-mediated end joining (TMEJ) [58]. Interestingly, POLQ-deficient

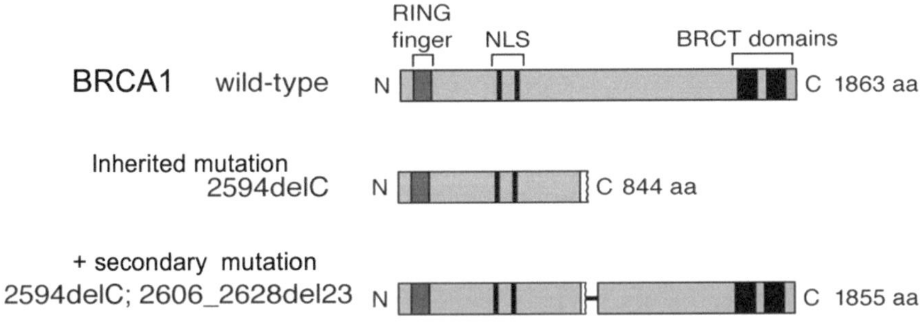

Fig. 2.2 An example of a secondary *BRCA1* mutation (reversion mutation) observed in recurrent platinum-resistant tumors of BRCA1 mutant ovarian cancer. (Adapted from [52]). Schematic representation of the BRCA1 proteins. In this tumor, a secondary *BRCA1* mutation (reversion mutation) cancels the frameshift caused by the germline (inherited) *BRCA1* mutation, allowing for the expression of a BRCA1 protein almost identical in length to the wild type (1855 amino acids)

cells accumulate post-replicative ssDNA gaps upon BRCA1/2 loss or PARP inhibitor treatment, suggesting a role of POLQ in mutagenic post-replicative gap sealing [59]. Other studies also suggest that persistence of ssDNA gaps underlies the synthetic lethality between BRCA1/2 and polθ [60, 61]. Polθ inhibitors, such as ART4215, have been developed [62, 63] and may have the potential to prevent the accumulation of reversion mutations. Furthermore, polθ is essential for cell survival in homologous-recombination-deficient cells, such as BRCA-deficient cells [64, 65], and homologous-recombination-deficient cells are sensitive to polθ inhibitors [62, 63]. In other words, BRCA-deficiency and polθ inhibition is a synthetic lethal combination. Thus, polθ inhibitors may serve an important role in cancer treatment and have gained great interest [58, 66].

When reversion mutations occur, both functions of BRCA1 and BRCA2, namely, homologous recombination [50, 51] and protection of replication forks [23], are restored. Since BRCA dysfunction is originally the cause of sensitivity to platinum and PARP inhibitors, it is logical for functional restoration to become a resistance mechanism.

In fact, *BRCA1* and *BRCA2* reversion mutations are clinically significant resistance mechanisms confirmed in numerous clinical cases [55, 56, 67–70]. *BRCA1/2* reversion mutations occur not only in ovarian cancer, but also in breast, pancreatic, prostate cancers and other cancers resistant to platinum and/or PARP inhibitors [71–79]. *BRCA1/2* reversion mutations (secondary mutations) are somatic mutations, but the primary *BRCA1/2* mutations preceding them are either germline or somatic in origin [70, 74]. *BRCA1/2* reversion mutations can be detected from circulating tumor DNA [70, 73, 75, 80–86]. However, caution should be exercised, because, theoretically, reversion mutations to wild type (back mutations) [66] could easily be missed in circulating tumor DNA. Multiple *BRCA1/2* reversion mutations can also be observed in resistant tumors or even in circulating tumor DNA in a single patient [67, 70, 75, 81, 86–92]. Furthermore, reversion mutations are observed when tumors with mutations in *RAD51B*, *RAD51C, RAD51D*, and *PALB2*, which control homologous recombination, become resistant to PARP inhibitors [68, 73, 93, 94]. Regarding reversion mutations of *BRCA1/2*, *RAD51C*, *RAD51D*, and *PALB2*, a database compiling them has been established (https://reversions.icr.ac.uk/) [55].

On the other hand, if the original *BRCA1/2* mutation is a very large deletion or structural abnormality, it is impossible to restore BRCA1/2 function with a reversion mutation; such *BRCA1/2* mutations have been found in ovarian cancer cases that have had long-term responses to PARP inhibitors [95, 96].

2.3 Partial Functional Restoration of BRCA1/2 by Utilizing Mutant (hypomorphic) *BRCA1/2* Alleles

In *BRCA1*-mutated tumors, residual functions of *BRCA1* mutant alleles may contribute to the acquisition of resistance to platinum and PARP inhibitors. The residual function of BRCA1.C61G mutant protein is implicated in resistance [97]. Additionally, in BRCA1 exon 11 mutant tumors, partially truncated BRCA1 lacking exon 11, generated through alternative splicing, is expressed and associated with resistance [98]. The BRCA1.5396 + 1C > A mutant protein is stabilized by HSP90 and involved in resistance [99]. There is an internal translation initiation site downstream of the frameshift mutation *BRCA1.185delAG*, where a slightly shorter BRCA1 protein with residual function is translated and involved in resistance [100, 101].

Similarly, amplification of the mutated *BRCA2* allele contributes to PARP inhibitor resistance in the *BRCA2*-mutated pancreatic cancer cell line, Capan-1, in the absence of reversion mutations [102].

2.4 Restoration of BRCA1 Expression in *BRCA1*-Methylated Tumors

In breast and ovarian cancers where BRCA1 expression is suppressed due to *BRCA1* promoter methylation, resistance to platinum and PARP inhibitors occurs through restoration of BRCA1 expression via promoter demethylation or by utilizing the promoters of genes involved in fusion with BRCA1, leading to its expression recovery [105, 106]. Similarly, in *RAD51C*-methylated ovarian cancer, restoration of RAD51C expression due to loss of *RAD51C* methylation can lead to PARP inhibitor resistance [107, 108].

2.5 Elevated RAD51 Protein Levels in BRCA2-Deficient Cancer Cells

An important function of BRCA2 is to replace RPA with RAD51 by recruiting RAD51 to the RPA-coated ssDNA generated by resection. Interestingly, elevated RAD51 expression in BRCA2-deficient cells leads to PARP inhibitor resistance. For example, it has been reported that loss of expression of E2F7, a transcriptional repressor of RAD51, in BRCA2-deficient cells results in increased RAD51 expression and PARP inhibitor resistance [103]. In addition, loss of the ubiquitin ligase HUWE1 in BRCA2-deficient cells increases the expression of RAD51 mRNA and RAD51 protein, leading to increased efficiency of homologous recombination and PARP inhibitor resistance [104].

2.6 Deficiency of 53BP1-Related Factors in BRCA1-Deficient Tumors

There are two well-known major methods for repairing DNA double-strand breaks: homologous recombination (HR) and non-homologous end joining (NHEJ). The balance between these two mechanisms is regulated by BRCA1 and 53BP1 (TP53BP1). BRCA1 promotes homologous recombination, while 53BP1 promotes non-homologous end joining [109]. In cases where homologous recombination is favored, it is necessary for single-strand DNA to be created by "resection" from the DNA double-strand break site in the $5' > 3'$ direction. In BRCA1-deficient cells, this resection step does not progress, preventing proper homologous recombination and resulting in sensitivity to PARP inhibitors. However, when 53BP1 is deficient in BRCA1-deficient cells, resection and homologous recombination are restored, leading to resistance to PARP inhibitors [110–114]. Factors that work together with 53BP1 (such as RIF1, REV7/MAD2L2/FANCV, Shieldin complex (RINN1, RINN2/FAM35A, RINN3), CST (CTC1-STN1-TEN1) complex, and DNA polymerase alpha) collectively form a barrier at the double-strand break site to prevent resection [109, 115–124]. BRCA1 overcomes this barrier to initiate resection [125]. BRCA1, when bound to BARD1, acts as a ubiquitin ligase, ubiquitinating histone H2A at K125/127/129. Ubiquitinated histone H2A is recognized by SMARCAD1, which induces sliding or removal of nucleosomes bound by 53BP1. As a result, the barrier is removed, allowing resection to occur [125]. When factors involved in the 53BP1 pathway (53BP1, RIF1, REV7, Shieldin complex, CST complex, DNA polymerase alpha, etc.) are deficient, the barrier that suppresses resection fails to function properly, allowing resection and homologous recombination to occur even in the absence of BRCA1, leading to resistance to PARP inhibitors. Additionally, overexpression of TRIP13, which inactivates REV7, in BRCA1-deficient cells also leads to PARP inhibitor resistance for similar reasons [126, 127]. On the other hand, BRCA2 is not critical for resection, and BRCA2-deficient cells do not become resistant to PARP inhibitors through these mechanisms. Interestingly, in BRCA2-deficient cells, loss of KAT5 (TIP60) promotes 53BP1 binding to DNA double-strand breaks and leads to PARP inhibitor resistance, suggesting that increasing NHEJ (rather than inhibiting NHEJ) may promote PARP inhibitor resistance in BRCA2-deficient cells [104].

Clinical evidence of inactivation of these 53BP1-related factors in clinical samples of PARP inhibitor resistant tumors is rather limited, but mutations in *53BP1 (TP53BP1)* and *RIF1* have been reported in a small number of cases with *BRCA1*-mutated PARP inhibitor-resistant breast cancer [128]. These mutations sometimes co-occur with *BRCA1* reversion mutations [128].

2.7 Restoration of Replication Fork Protection

In BRCA1/2-deficient cells, the protection of replication forks is also diminished. Restoration of either homologous recombination or replication fork protection leads to resistance to PARP inhibitors [129, 130]. When DNA replication is stressed by agents like platinum or PARP inhibitors, replication forks stall, leading to a phenomenon known as fork reversal [131–133]. In the absence of functioning BRCA1 or BRCA2, reversed forks serve as initiation points for degradation of nascent DNA strands by a nuclease called MRE11 [23]. Additionally, in the absence of functioning BRCA2, cleavage of replication fork DNA occurs by a nuclease called MUS81 [134]. These processes contribute to replication fork instability and sensitivity to platinum and PARP inhibitors.

The recovery of replication fork protection (stabilization) is a mechanism for resistance to platinum and PARP inhibitors [129]. Since fork reversal precedes DNA degradation at forks, suppression of the expression of factors involved in fork reversal, such as SMARCAL1, ZRANB3, and HLTF, stabilizes replication forks and confers cisplatin and PARP inhibitor resistance even in BRCA1/2-deficient cells [132, 135]. Depletion of RADX, a single-stranded DNA-binding protein that negatively regulates RAD51, restores replication fork protection in BRCA2-deficient cells, leading to PARP inhibitor resistance [136]. Furthermore, depletion of PTIP (PAXIP1), MLL3/4, and PARP1, which are involved in recruitment of MRE11 to replication forks, or depletion of CHD4 in BRCA2-deficient cells, protects replication forks and confers resistance to platinum and PARP inhibitors [129, 137]. Similarly, loss of the mono-ADP-ribosyltransferase PARP14, which is a critical cofactor of MRE11, suppresses MRE11 engagement on nascent DNA and MRE11-mediated fork degradation in BRCA-deficient cells, and causes chemoresistance to cisplatin and PARP inhibitors [138]. Since EZH2 is involved in recruiting MUS81, depletion of EZH2 in BRCA2-deficient cells also protects replication forks, leading to resistance to platinum and PARP inhibitors [134]. Furthermore, loss of MED12 leads to TGFβ activation, which results in restoration of both homologous recombination and replication fork stability and resistance to cisplatin and PARP inhibitors [139].

There is still limited evidence that these drug resistance mechanisms are clinically relevant. For example, mutations in *PAXIP1/PTIP* have been reported in a small number of clinical cases with *BRCA2*-mutated breast cancer [128]. These mutations sometimes co-occur with *BRCA2* reversion mutations [128].

2.8 ssDNA Gap Suppression

BRCA1 and BRCA2 are involved in replication gap inhibition (ssDNA gap inhibition), and this function of BRCA1/2 is increasingly recognized as important for PARP inhibitor resistance, since accumulation of ssDNA gaps, rather than double-strand breaks or degradation of stalled replication forks, in BRCA-deficient cells has been shown to correlate with chemosensitivity to PARP inhibitors and platinum compounds [25–30, 133, 138, 140, 141].

ssDNA gaps can be generated on the lagging strands when the Okazaki fragment processing is perturbed [142]. PARP1 is implicated in the detection and processing of unligated Okazaki fragments during DNA replication [143, 144]. In cells treated with PARP inhibitor, unligated Okazaki fragments persist and fork speed becomes higher, leading to increased genome instability and replication conflicts in the subsequent S phase [143–145].

During perturbed DNA replication with replication obstacles, replication obstacles can be tolerated by three different pathways to resume replication fork progression: translesion synthesis, template switching or fork reversal, and repriming [146]. Primase-polymerase (PRIMPOL)-mediated repriming of DNA synthesis also results in ssDNA gap generation [147]. ssDNA gaps can be expanded by the MRE11 and EXO1 nucleases [141, 148, 149], and the gap expansion promotes their conversion into double-strand breaks through the endonucleolytic activity of MRE11 on the parental strand at the ssDNA gap region [148, 149]. ssDNA gaps are filled by two distinct mechanisms: RAD18, PCNA monoubiquitination, and REV1-POLζ promote gap filling in G2 phase of the cell cycle, while UBC13, RAD51, and REV1-POLζ promote gap filling in S phase [141, 147]. BRCA1 and BRCA2 promote gap filling by limiting MRE11 activity [141]. Furthermore, BRCA2 associates with MCM10 and this association suppresses PRIMPOL-mediated repriming and ssDNA gap formation [29].Thus, BRCA1 and BRCA2 are involved in suppression of ssDNA gap generation, and diminished ability to suppress ssDNA gap generation can be the cause of PARP inhibitor sensitivity of BRCA1/2-deficient cells. If these cells restore the ability to suppress ssDNA gap, it may lead to PARP inhibitor resistance.

2.9 Increased Extracellular Drug Efflux via p-Glycoprotein

p-Glycoprotein (ABCB1/MDR1) is a transporter that pumps drugs out of cells. Olaparib, niraparib, talazoparib, and rucaparib are expelled from cells via p-glycoprotein, so an increase in p-glycoprotein expression can lead to resistance to these PARP inhibitors [150–152]. On the other hand, veliparib and AZD2461 are not robust substrates for p-glycoprotein [153]. When increased p-glycoprotein expression is the cause of resistance, sensitivity can be restored by using p-glycoprotein inhibitor tariquidar [150]. It has been reported that increased expression of p-glycoprotein was observed in 15% of ovarian cancer cases participating in clinical trials using PARP inhibitors after other drug therapies [68], suggesting a potential involvement of p-glycoprotein in PARP inhibitor resistance in clinical settings. On the other hand, p-glycoprotein is not involved in cisplatin resistance, at least in ovarian cancer cell lines [154].

2.10 *PARP1* Mutations

A *PARP1* mutation (*PARP1 p.R591C*) that prevents PARP1 from being trapped in DNA can cause PARP inhibitor resistance, and one clinical case of ovarian cancer with this mutation has been reported [155].

2.11 Phosphorylation of PARP1 by c-Met

The receptor tyrosine kinase c-Met phosphorylates Tyr907 of PARP1, increasing PARP1 activity and decreasing its binding with PARP inhibitors. Therefore, c-Met can potentially induce PARP inhibitor resistance [156].

2.12 Loss of Poly(ADP-ribose) Glycohydrolase (PARG)

PARG works in opposition to PARP by removing poly(ADP-ribose), and its deficiency contributes to PARP inhibitor resistance [114, 157]. Since PARP inhibition by PARP inhibitors is not 100% effective, in the absence of PARG, the remaining PARP activity leads to increased poly(ADP-ribose) formation. This reduces the trapping of PARP1 to DNA and allows for the repair of single-strand breaks. In some portions of triple-negative breast cancer and ovarian cancer tissues, PARG expression may not be detectable, suggesting a potential for cancer cells in those sites to develop PARP inhibitor resistance [157]. Interestingly, restoration of PARP signaling via PARG loss is a dominant resistance mechanism of PARP inhibitors in *Brca2*-knockout tumors in which genetic reversion of *Brca2* mutation is impossible [114].

2.13 Overexpression of ALC1

ALC1 (amplified in liver cancer 1), which performs chromatin remodeling, has functions to remove trapped PARP and to protect PARP from PARG-mediated depoly(ADP-ribosyl)ation [158–161]. Deletion of ALC1 increases sensitivity to PARP inhibitors. Overexpression of ALC1 in BRCA1/2-deficient cells decreases sensitivity to PARP inhibitors [158], suggesting a possible role of ALC1 in resistance to PARP inhibitor.

2.14 Other Mechanisms

SLFN11 is a factor involved in platinum and PARP inhibitor resistance [162, 163]. In the presence of replication stress, SLFN11 binds to chromatin and irreversibly arrests DNA replication, enhancing the efficacy of chemotherapy. Conversely, loss or reduced expression of SLFN11 results in PARP inhibitor resistance [162, 163]. In clinical trials of PARP inhibitors for ovarian cancer, decreased expression of SLFN11 has been reported in 7% of cases [68]. SLFN11-deficient cells depend on ATR for survival in the presence of PARP inhibitors, suggesting that ATR inhibitors may be effective [162].

Other diverse resistance mechanisms have been proposed: phosphorylation of ribosomal protein S6 is involved in PARP inhibitor resistance in BRCA1 mutant breast cancer cells [164]. Ovarian cancer cells with non-homologous end linkage defects become resistant to PARP inhibitors [165]. A microRNA (miR-622) targeting the Ku complex involved in non-homologous end joining restores homologous recombination in BRCA1-deficient cells and causes PARP inhibitor resistance [166]. Stabilization of FZD10 mRNA by adenosine-N6-methylation enhances the Wnt/β-catenin pathway, leading to PARP inhibitor resistance [167].

New mechanisms of PARP inhibitor resistance continue to be reported, and their clinical significance is expected to become clearer in the future. The current major challenge is to establish effective treatments for resistant tumors and strategies to prevent resistance. For information on combinations of PARP inhibitors with other agents tested for ovarian cancer, please refer to other reviews [17, 49, 168]. Broadly categorized, these combinations include (1) PARP inhibitors with conventional chemotherapy agents (such as carboplatin, paclitaxel), (2) PARP inhibitors with antiangiogenic agents, (3) PARP inhibitors with immune checkpoint inhibitors, (4) PARP inhibitors with other agents targeting DNA damage response (such as ATR inhibitors, Wee1 inhibitors, Chk1/2 inhibitors, CDK12 inhibitors), and (5) PARP inhibitors with polθ inhibitors.

However, ovarian cancer exhibits high intratumoral heterogeneity [169], and multiple resistance mechanisms may operate within a single patient's tumor [85, 128, 170]. Therefore, treatment of PARP inhibitor-resistant tumors may also not work with a simple strategy, and further studies are awaited.

Conflict of Interest TT has received speaker fees from AstraZeneca.

References

1. Groelly FJ, Fawkes M, Dagg RA, Blackford AN, Tarsounas M. Targeting DNA damage response pathways in cancer. Nat Rev Cancer. 2023;23:78–94.
2. Fong PC, Boss DS, Yap TA, Tutt A, Wu P, Mergui-Roelvink M, et al. Inhibition of poly(ADP-Ribose) polymerase in tumors from BRCA mutation carriers. N Engl J Med. 2009;361:123–34.

3. Fong PC, Yap TA, Boss DS, Carden CP, Mergui-Roelvink M, Gourley C, et al. Poly(ADP)-ribose polymerase inhibition: frequent durable responses in BRCA carrier ovarian cancer correlating with platinum-free interval. J Clin Oncol. 2010;28:2512–9.
4. Audeh MW, Carmichael J, Penson RT, Friedlander M, Powell B, Bell-McGuinn KM, et al. Oral poly(ADP-ribose) polymerase inhibitor olaparib in patients with BRCA1 or BRCA2 mutations and recurrent ovarian cancer: a proof-of-concept trial. Lancet. 2010;376:245–51.
5. Ledermann J, Harter P, Gourley C, Friedlander M, Vergote I, Rustin G, et al. Olaparib maintenance therapy in patients with platinum-sensitive relapsed serous ovarian cancer: a preplanned retrospective analysis of outcomes by BRCA status in a randomised phase 2 trial. Lancet Oncol. 2014;15:852–61.
6. Ledermann JA, Harter P, Gourley C, Friedlander M, Vergote I, Rustin G, et al. Overall survival in patients with platinum-sensitive recurrent serous ovarian cancer receiving olaparib maintenance monotherapy: an updated analysis from a randomised, placebo-controlled, double-blind, phase 2 trial. Lancet Oncol. 2016;17:1579–89.
7. Moore K, Colombo N, Scambia G, Kim B-G, Oaknin A, Friedlander M, et al. Maintenance olaparib in patients with newly diagnosed advanced ovarian cancer. N Engl J Med. 2018;379:2495–505.
8. Tutt A, Robson M, Garber JE, Domchek SM, Audeh MW, Weitzel JN, et al. Oral poly(ADP-ribose) polymerase inhibitor olaparib in patients with BRCA1 or BRCA2 mutations and advanced breast cancer: a proof-of-concept trial. Lancet. 2010;376:235–44.
9. Robson M, Im S-A, Senkus E, Xu B, Domchek SM, Masuda N, et al. Olaparib for metastatic breast cancer in patients with a germline BRCA mutation. N Engl J Med. 2017;377:523–33.
10. Tutt ANJ, Garber JE, Kaufman B, Viale G, Fumagalli D, Rastogi P, et al. Adjuvant olaparib for patients with BRCA1 – or BRCA2 -mutated breast cancer. N Engl J Med. 2021;384:2394–405.
11. Litton JK, Rugo HS, Ettl J, Hurvitz SA, Gonçalves A, Lee K-H, et al. Talazoparib in patients with advanced breast cancer and a germline BRCA mutation. N Engl J Med. 2018;379:753–63.
12. Golan T, Hammel P, Reni M, Van Cutsem E, Macarulla T, Hall MJ, et al. Maintenance olaparib for germline BRCA -mutated metastatic pancreatic cancer. N Engl J Med. 2019;381:317–27.
13. Mateo J, Carreira S, Sandhu S, Miranda S, Mossop H, Perez-Lopez R, et al. DNA-repair defects and olaparib in metastatic prostate cancer. N Engl J Med. 2015;373:1697–708.
14. Abida W, Patnaik A, Campbell D, Shapiro J, Bryce AH, McDermott R, et al. Rucaparib in men with metastatic castration-resistant prostate cancer harboring a BRCA1 or BRCA2 gene alteration. J Clin Oncol. 2020;38:3763–72.
15. De Bono J, Mateo J, Fizazi K, Saad F, Shore N, Sandhu S, et al. Olaparib for metastatic castration-resistant prostate cancer. N Engl J Med. 2020;382:2091–102.
16. Hussain M, Mateo J, Fizazi K, Saad F, Shore N, Sandhu S, et al. Survival with olaparib in metastatic castration-resistant prostate cancer. N Engl J Med. 2020;383:2345–57.
17. Chiappa M, Guffanti F, Bertoni F, Colombo I, Damia G. Overcoming PARPi resistance: preclinical and clinical evidence in ovarian cancer. Drug Resist Updat. 2021;55:100744.
18. Momozawa Y, Sasai R, Usui Y, Shiraishi K, Iwasaki Y, Taniyama Y, et al. Expansion of cancer risk profile for BRCA1 and BRCA2 pathogenic variants. JAMA Oncol. 2022;8:871.
19. Sawyer SL, Tian L, Kähkönen M, Schwartzentruber J, Kircher M, University of Washington Centre for Mendelian Genomics, et al. Biallelic mutations in BRCA1 cause a new fanconi anemia subtype. Cancer Discov. 2015;5:135–42.
20. Howlett NG, Taniguchi T, Olson S, Cox B, Waisfisz Q, De Die-Smulders C, et al. Biallelic inactivation of BRCA2 in fanconi anemia. Science. 2002;297:606–9.
21. Moynahan ME, Chiu JW, Koller BH, Jasin M. Brca1 controls homology-directed DNA repair. Mol Cell. 1999;4:511–8.
22. Moynahan ME, Pierce AJ, Jasin M. BRCA2 is required for homology-directed repair of chromosomal breaks. Mol Cell. 2001;7:263–72.

23. Schlacher K, Christ N, Siaud N, Egashira A, Wu H, Jasin M. Double-strand break repair-independent role for BRCA2 in blocking stalled replication fork degradation by MRE11. Cell. 2011;145:529–42.
24. Schlacher K, Wu H, Jasin M. A distinct replication fork protection pathway connects Fanconi anemia tumor suppressors to RAD51-BRCA1/2. Cancer Cell. 2012;22:106–16.
25. Cong K, Peng M, Kousholt AN, Lee WTC, Lee S, Nayak S, et al. Replication gaps are a key determinant of PARP inhibitor synthetic lethality with BRCA deficiency. Mol Cell. 2021;81:3128–3144.e7.
26. Cantor SB. Revisiting the BRCA-pathway through the lens of replication gap suppression. DNA Repair. 2021;107:103209.
27. Vugic D, Dumoulin I, Martin C, Minello A, Alvaro-Aranda L, Gomez-Escudero J, et al. Replication gap suppression depends on the double-strand DNA binding activity of BRCA2. Nat Commun. 2023;14:446.
28. Panzarino NJ, Krais JJ, Cong K, Peng M, Mosqueda M, Nayak SU, et al. Replication gaps underlie BRCA deficiency and therapy response. Cancer Res. 2021;81:1388–97.
29. Kang Z, Fu P, Alcivar AL, Fu H, Redon C, Foo TK, et al. BRCA2 associates with MCM10 to suppress PRIMPOL-mediated repriming and single-stranded gap formation after DNA damage. Nat Commun. 2021;12:5966.
30. Simoneau A, Xiong R, Zou L. The trans cell cycle effects of PARP inhibitors underlie their selectivity toward BRCA1/2-deficient cells. Genes Dev. 2021;35:1271–89.
31. Lim PX, Zaman M, Feng W, Jasin M. BRCA2 promotes genomic integrity and therapy resistance primarily through its role in homology-directed repair. Mol Cell. 2024;84:447–462.e10.
32. Dibitetto D, Rottenberg S. DNA repair, gap suppression, or fork protection: BRCA2 needs a break! Mol Cell. 2024;84:409–10.
33. Feng W, Jasin M. BRCA2 suppresses replication stress-induced mitotic and G1 abnormalities through homologous recombination. Nat Commun. 2017;8:525.
34. Semlow DR, Walter JC. Mechanisms of Vertebrate DNA Interstrand Cross-Link Repair. Annu Rev Biochem. 2021;90:107–35.
35. Lord CJ, Tutt ANJ, Ashworth A. Synthetic lethality and cancer therapy: lessons learned from the development of PARP inhibitors. Annu Rev Med. 2015;66:455–70.
36. Dhillon KK, Bajrami I, Taniguchi T, Lord CJ. Synthetic lethality: the road to novel therapies for breast cancer. Endocr Relat Cancer. 2016;23:T39–55.
37. Farmer H, McCabe N, Lord CJ, Tutt ANJ, Johnson DA, Richardson TB, et al. Targeting the DNA repair defect in BRCA mutant cells as a therapeutic strategy. Nature. 2005;434:917–21.
38. Bryant HE, Schultz N, Thomas HD, Parker KM, Flower D, Lopez E, et al. Specific killing of BRCA2-deficient tumours with inhibitors of poly(ADP-ribose) polymerase. 2005;434.
39. Murai J, Huang SN, Das BB, Renaud A, Zhang Y, Doroshow JH, et al. Trapping of PARP1 and PARP2 by clinical PARP inhibitors. Cancer Res. 2012;72:5588–99.
40. Murai J, Huang S-YN, Renaud A, Zhang Y, Ji J, Takeda S, et al. Stereospecific PARP trapping by BMN 673 and comparison with Olaparib and Rucaparib. Mol Cancer Ther. 2014;13:433–43.
41. Krastev DB, Wicks AJ, Lord CJ. PARP inhibitors – trapped in a toxic love affair. Cancer Res. 2021;81:5605–7.
42. Turner N, Tutt A, Ashworth A. Hallmarks of “BRCAness” in sporadic cancers. Nat Rev Cancer. 2004;4:814–9.
43. Lord CJ, Ashworth A. BRCAness revisited. Nat Rev Cancer. 2016;16:110–20.
44. Byrum AK, Vindigni A, Mosammaparast N. Defining and modulating ‘BRCAness’. Trends Cell Biol. 2019;29:740–51.
45. Konstantinopoulos PA, Ceccaldi R, Shapiro GI, D’Andrea AD. Homologous recombination deficiency: exploiting the fundamental vulnerability of ovarian cancer. Cancer Discov. 2015;5:1137–54.

46. González-Martín A, Pothuri B, Vergote I, DePont Christensen R, Graybill W, Mirza MR, et al. Niraparib in patients with newly diagnosed advanced ovarian cancer. N Engl J Med. 2019;381:2391–402.
47. Mirza MR, Monk BJ, Herrstedt J, Oza AM, Mahner S, Redondo A, et al. Niraparib maintenance therapy in platinum-sensitive, recurrent ovarian cancer. N Engl J Med. 2016;375:2154–64.
48. Jackson LM, Moldovan G-L. Mechanisms of PARP1 inhibitor resistance and their implications for cancer treatment. NAR Cancer. 2022;4:zcac042.
49. Collet L, Hanvic B, Turinetto M, Treilleux I, Chopin N, Le Saux O, et al. BRCA1/2 alterations and reversion mutations in the area of PARP inhibitors in high grade ovarian cancer: state of the art and forthcoming challenges. Front Oncol. 2024;14:1354427.
50. Sakai W, Swisher EM, Karlan BY, Agarwal MK, Higgins J, Friedman C, et al. Secondary mutations as a mechanism of cisplatin resistance in BRCA2-mutated cancers. Nature. 2008;451:1116–20.
51. Edwards SL, Brough R, Lord CJ, Natrajan R, Vatcheva R, Levine DA, et al. Resistance to therapy caused by intragenic deletion in BRCA2. Nature. 2008;451:1111–5.
52. Swisher EM, Sakai W, Karlan BY, Wurz K, Urban N, Taniguchi T. Secondary BRCA1 mutations in BRCA1 -mutated ovarian carcinomas with platinum resistance. Cancer Res. 2008;68:2581–6.
53. Sakai W, Swisher EM, Jacquemont C, Chandramohan KV, Couch FJ, Langdon SP, et al. Functional restoration of BRCA2 Protein by secondary BRCA2 mutations in BRCA2 -mutated ovarian carcinoma. Cancer Res. 2009;69:6381–6.
54. Dhillon KK, Swisher EM, Taniguchi T. Secondary mutations of BRCA1/2 and drug resistance. Cancer Sci. 2011;102:663–9.
55. Pettitt SJ, Frankum JR, Punta M, Lise S, Alexander J, Chen Y, et al. Clinical BRCA1/2 reversion analysis identifies hotspot mutations and predicted neoantigens associated with therapy resistance. Cancer Discov. 2020;10:1475–88.
56. Tobalina L, Armenia J, Irving E, O'Connor MJ, Forment JV. A meta-analysis of reversion mutations in BRCA genes identifies signatures of DNA end-joining repair mechanisms driving therapy resistance. Ann Oncol. 2021;32:103–12.
57. Wyatt DW, Feng W, Conlin MP, Yousefzadeh MJ, Roberts SA, Mieczkowski P, et al. Essential roles for polymerase θ-mediated end joining in the repair of chromosome breaks. Mol Cell. 2016;63:662–73.
58. Schrempf A, Slyskova J, Loizou JI. Targeting the DNA repair enzyme polymerase θ in cancer therapy. Trends Cancer. 2021;7:98–111.
59. Belan O, Sebald M, Adamowicz M, Anand R, Vancevska A, Neves J, et al. POLQ seals post-replicative ssDNA gaps to maintain genome stability in BRCA-deficient cancer cells. Mol Cell. 2022;82:4664–4680.e9.
60. Schrempf A, Bernardo S, Arasa Verge EA, Ramirez Otero MA, Wilson J, Kirchhofer D, et al. POLθ processes ssDNA gaps and promotes replication fork progression in BRCA1-deficient cells. Cell Rep. 2022;41:111716.
61. Mann A, Ramirez-Otero MA, De Antoni A, Hanthi YW, Sannino V, Baldi G, et al. POLθ prevents MRE11-NBS1-CtIP-dependent fork breakage in the absence of BRCA2/RAD51 by filling lagging-strand gaps. Mol Cell. 2022;82:4218–4231.e8.
62. Zhou J, Gelot C, Pantelidou C, Li A, Yücel H, Davis RE, et al. A first-in-class polymerase theta inhibitor selectively targets homologous-recombination-deficient tumors. Nat Cancer. 2021;2:598–610.
63. Zatreanu D, Robinson HMR, Alkhatib O, Boursier M, Finch H, Geo L, et al. Polθ inhibitors elicit BRCA-gene synthetic lethality and target PARP inhibitor resistance. Nat Commun. 2021;12:3636.
64. Ceccaldi R, Liu JC, Amunugama R, Hajdu I, Primack B, Petalcorin MIR, et al. Homologous-recombination-deficient tumours are dependent on Polθ-mediated repair. Nature. 2015;518:258–62.

65. Mateos-Gomez PA, Gong F, Nair N, Miller KM, Lazzerini-Denchi E, Sfeir A. Mammalian polymerase θ promotes alternative NHEJ and suppresses recombination. Nature. 2015;518:254–7.
66. Pismataro MC, Astolfi A, Barreca ML, Pacetti M, Schenone S, Bandiera T, et al. Small molecules targeting DNA polymerase theta (POLθ) as promising synthetic lethal agents for precision cancer therapy. J Med Chem. 2023;66:6498–522.
67. Patch A-M, Christie EL, Etemadmoghadam D, Garsed DW, George J, Fereday S, et al. Whole–genome characterization of chemoresistant ovarian cancer. Nature. 2015;521:489–94.
68. Lheureux S, Oaknin A, Garg S, Bruce JP, Madariaga A, Dhani NC, et al. EVOLVE: a multicenter open-label single-arm clinical and translational phase II Trial of Cediranib plus Olaparib for ovarian cancer after PARP inhibition progression. Clin Cancer Res. 2020;26:4206–15.
69. Norquist B, Wurz KA, Pennil CC, Garcia R, Gross J, Sakai W, et al. Secondary somatic mutations restoring BRCA1/2 predict chemotherapy resistance in hereditary ovarian carcinomas. J Clin Oncol. 2011;29:3008–15.
70. Lin KK, Harrell MI, Oza AM, Oaknin A, Ray-Coquard I, Tinker AV, et al. BRCA reversion mutations in circulating tumor DNA predict primary and acquired resistance to the PARP inhibitor Rucaparib in high-grade ovarian carcinoma. Cancer Discov. 2019;9:210–9.
71. Afghahi A, Timms KM, Vinayak S, Jensen KC, Kurian AW, Carlson RW, et al. Tumor BRCA1 reversion mutation arising during neoadjuvant platinum-based chemotherapy in triple-negative breast cancer is associated with therapy resistance. Clin Cancer Res. 2017;23:3365–70.
72. Pishvaian MJ, Biankin AV, Bailey P, Chang DK, Laheru D, Wolfgang CL, et al. BRCA2 secondary mutation-mediated resistance to platinum and PARP inhibitor-based therapy in pancreatic cancer. Br J Cancer. 2017;116:1021–6.
73. Brown TJ, Yablonovitch A, Till JE, Yen J, Kiedrowski LA, Hood R, et al. The clinical implications of reversions in patients with advanced pancreatic cancer and pathogenic variants in BRCA1, BRCA2, or PALB2 after progression on Rucaparib. Clin Cancer Res. 2023;29:5207–16.
74. Carneiro BA, Collier KA, Nagy RJ, Pamarthy S, Sagar V, Fairclough S, et al. Acquired resistance to poly (ADP-ribose) polymerase inhibitor olaparib in BRCA2 -associated prostate cancer resulting From Biallelic BRCA2 reversion mutations restores both germline and somatic loss-of-function mutations. JCO Precis Oncol. 2018:1–8.
75. Walmsley CS, Jonsson P, Cheng ML, McBride S, Kaeser C, Vargas HA, et al. Convergent evolution of BRCA2 reversion mutations under therapeutic pressure by PARP inhibition and platinum chemotherapy. Npj Precis Oncol. 2024;8:34.
76. Nakamura K, Hayashi H, Kawano R, Ishikawa M, Aimono E, Mizuno T, et al. BRCA1/2 reversion mutations in a pan-cancer cohort. Cancer Sci. 2024;115:635–47.
77. Darabi S, Braxton DR, Xiu J, Carneiro BA, Swensen J, Antonarakis ES, et al. BRCA1/2 reversion mutations in patients treated with poly ADP-ribose polymerase (PARP) inhibitors or platinum agents. Medicina (Mex). 2022;58:1818.
78. Murciano-Goroff YR, Schram AM, Rosen EY, Won H, Gong Y, Noronha AM, et al. Reversion mutations in germline BRCA1/2-mutant tumors reveal a BRCA-mediated phenotype in non-canonical histologies. Nat Commun. 2022;13:7182.
79. Zong H, Zhang J, Xu Z, Pan J-N, Wang R, Han J, et al. Comprehensive analysis of somatic reversion mutations in homologous recombination repair (HRR) genes in a large cohort of chinese pan-cancer patients. J Cancer. 2022;13:1119–29.
80. Christie EL, Fereday S, Doig K, Pattnaik S, Dawson S-J, Bowtell DDL. Reversion of BRCA1/2 germline mutations detected in circulating tumor DNA from patients with high-grade serous ovarian cancer. J Clin Oncol. 2017;35:1274–80.
81. Quigley D, Alumkal JJ, Wyatt AW, Kothari V, Foye A, Lloyd P, et al. Analysis of circulating cell-free DNA identifies multiclonal heterogeneity of BRCA2 reversion mutations associated with resistance to PARP inhibitors. Cancer Discov. 2017;7:999–1005.

82. Mayor P, Gay LM, Lele S, Elvin JA. BRCA1 reversion mutation acquired after treatment identified by liquid biopsy. Gynecol Oncol Rep. 2017;21:57–60.
83. Weigelt B, Comino-Méndez I, De Bruijn I, Tian L, Meisel JL, García-Murillas I, et al. Diverse BRCA1 and BRCA2 reversion mutations in circulating cell-free DNA of therapy-resistant breast or ovarian cancer. Clin Cancer Res. 2017;23:6708–20.
84. Lheureux S, Prokopec SD, Oldfield LE, Gonzalez-Ochoa E, Bruce JP, Wong D, et al. Identifying mechanisms of resistance by circulating tumor DNA in EVOLVE, a phase II trial of Cediranib plus Olaparib for ovarian cancer at time of parp inhibitor progression. Clin Cancer Res. 2023;29:3706–16.
85. Kim Y-N, Shim Y, Seo J, Choi Z, Lee YJ, Shin S, et al. Investigation of PARP inhibitor resistance based on serially collected circulating tumor DNA in patients with BRCA -mutated ovarian cancer. Clin Cancer Res. 2023;29:2725–34.
86. Sivakumar S, Jin DX, Tukachinsky H, Murugesan K, McGregor K, Danziger N, et al. Tissue and liquid biopsy profiling reveal convergent tumor evolution and therapy evasion in breast cancer. Nat Commun. 2022;13:7495.
87. Loehr A, Hussain A, Patnaik A, Bryce AH, Castellano D, Font A, et al. Emergence of BRCA reversion mutations in patients with metastatic castration-resistant prostate cancer after treatment with Rucaparib. Eur Urol. 2023;83:200–9.
88. Sorrells S, McKinnon KE, McBratney A, Sumey C. Longitudinal and multi-tissue molecular diagnostics track somatic BRCA2 reversion mutations that correct the open reading frame of germline alteration upon clinical relapse. NPJ Genomic Med. 2021;6:17.
89. Jacob SL, Kiedrowski LA, Chae YK. The dynamic landscape of BRCA1 reversion mutations from indel to SNV in a patient with ovarian cancer treated with PARP-inhibitors and immunotherapy. Heliyon. 2020;6:e03841.
90. Tao H, Liu S, Huang D, Han X, Wu X, Shao YW, et al. Acquired multiple secondary BRCA2 mutations upon PARPi resistance in a metastatic pancreatic cancer patient harboring a BRCA2 germline mutation.
91. Vidula N, Rich TA, Sartor O, Yen J, Hardin A, Nance T, et al. Routine plasma-based genotyping to comprehensively detect germline, somatic, and reversion brca mutations among patients with advanced solid tumors. Clin Cancer Res. 2020;26:2546–55.
92. McFarland TR, Tandar CE, Agarwal N, Swami U. Emergence of polyclonal BRCA2 reversions following PARP inhibitor treatment: An illustrative case report. Cancer Treat Res Commun. 2021;29:100480.
93. Kondrashova O, Nguyen M, Shield-Artin K, Tinker AV, Teng NNH, Harrell MI, et al. Secondary somatic mutations restoring RAD51C and RAD51D associated with acquired resistance to the PARP inhibitor Rucaparib in high-grade ovarian carcinoma. Cancer Discov. 2017;7:984–98.
94. Goodall J, Mateo J, Yuan W, Mossop H, Porta N, Miranda S, et al. Circulating cell-free DNA to guide prostate cancer treatment with PARP inhibition. Cancer Discov. 2017;7:1006–17.
95. Swisher EM, Kristeleit RS, Oza AM, Tinker AV, Ray-Coquard I, Oaknin A, et al. Characterization of patients with long-term responses to rucaparib treatment in recurrent ovarian cancer. Gynecol Oncol. 2021;163:490–7.
96. Randall M, Burgess K, Buckingham L, Usha L. Exceptional response to Olaparib in a patient with recurrent ovarian cancer and an entire BRCA1 germline gene deletion. J Natl Compr Cancer Netw. 2020;18:223–8.
97. Drost R, Bouwman P, Rottenberg S, Boon U, Schut E, Klarenbeek S, et al. BRCA1 RING function is essential for tumor suppression but dispensable for therapy resistance. Cancer Cell. 2011;20:797–809.
98. Wang Y, Bernhardy AJ, Cruz C, Krais JJ, Nacson J, Nicolas E, et al. The BRCA1-Δ11q alternative splice isoform bypasses germline mutations and promotes therapeutic resistance to PARP inhibition and cisplatin. Cancer Res. 2016;76:2778–90.

99. Johnson N, Johnson SF, Yao W, Li Y-C, Choi Y-E, Bernhardy AJ, et al. Stabilization of mutant BRCA1 protein confers PARP inhibitor and platinum resistance. Proc Natl Acad Sci. 2013;110:17041–6.
100. Drost R, Dhillon KK, Van Der Gulden H, Van Der Heijden I, Brandsma I, Cruz C, et al. BRCA1185delAG tumors may acquire therapy resistance through expression of RING-less BRCA1. J Clin Invest. 2016;126:2903–18.
101. Wang Y, Krais JJ, Bernhardy AJ, Nicolas E, Cai KQ, Harrell MI, et al. RING domain–deficient BRCA1 promotes PARP inhibitor and platinum resistance. J Clin Invest. 2016;126:3145–57.
102. Park PH, Yamamoto TM, Li H, Alcivar AL, Xia B, Wang Y, et al. Amplification of the mutation-carrying BRCA2 allele promotes RAD51 loading and PARP inhibitor resistance in the absence of reversion mutations. Mol Cancer Ther. 2020;19:602–13.
103. Clements KE, Thakar T, Nicolae CM, Liang X, Wang H-G, Moldovan G-L. Loss of E2F7 confers resistance to poly-ADP-ribose polymerase (PARP) inhibitors in BRCA2-deficient cells. Nucleic Acids Res. 2018;46:8898–907.
104. Clements KE, Schleicher EM, Thakar T, Hale A, Dhoonmoon A, Tolman NJ, et al. Identification of regulators of poly-ADP-ribose polymerase inhibitor response through complementary CRISPR knockout and activation screens. Nat Commun. 2020;11:6118.
105. Moschetta M, George A, Kaye SB, Banerjee S. BRCA somatic mutations and epigenetic BRCA modifications in serous ovarian cancer. Ann Oncol. 2016;27:1449–55.
106. Ter Brugge P, Kristel P, Van Der Burg E, Boon U, De Maaker M, Lips E, et al. Mechanisms of therapy resistance in patient-derived xenograft models of BRCA1-deficient breast cancer. J Natl Cancer Inst. 2016;108:djw148.
107. Nesic K, Kondrashova O, Hurley RM, McGehee CD, Vandenberg CJ, Ho G-Y, et al. Acquired RAD51C promoter methylation loss causes PARP inhibitor resistance in high-grade serous ovarian carcinoma. Cancer Res. 2021;81:4709–22.
108. Hurley RM, McGehee CD, Nesic K, Correia C, Weiskittel TM, Kelly RL, et al. Characterization of a RAD51C -silenced high-grade serous ovarian cancer model during development of PARP inhibitor resistance. NAR Cancer. 2021;3:zcab028.
109. Shibata A. Regulation of repair pathway choice at two-ended DNA double-strand breaks. Mutat Res Mol Mech Mutagen. 2017;803–805:51–5.
110. Bunting SF, Callén E, Wong N, Chen H-T, Polato F, Gunn A, et al. 53BP1 inhibits homologous recombination in Brca1-deficient cells by blocking resection of DNA breaks. Cell. 2010;141:243–54.
111. Cao L, Xu X, Bunting SF, Liu J, Wang R-H, Cao LL, et al. A selective requirement for 53BP1 in the biological response to genomic instability induced by Brca1 deficiency. Mol Cell. 2009;35:534–41.
112. Bouwman P, Aly A, Escandell JM, Pieterse M, Bartkova J, Van Der Gulden H, et al. 53BP1 loss rescues BRCA1 deficiency and is associated with triple-negative and BRCA-mutated breast cancers. Nat Struct Mol Biol. 2010;17:688–95.
113. Jaspers JE, Kersbergen A, Boon U, Sol W, Van Deemter L, Zander SA, et al. Loss of 53BP1 causes PARP inhibitor resistance in Brca1 -mutated mouse mammary tumors. Cancer Discov. 2013;3:68–81.
114. Bhin J, Paes Dias M, Gogola E, Rolfs F, Piersma SR, De Bruijn R, et al. Multi-omics analysis reveals distinct non-reversion mechanisms of PARPi resistance in BRCA1- versus BRCA2-deficient mammary tumors. Cell Rep. 2023;42:112538.
115. Chapman JR, Barral P, Vannier J-B, Borel V, Steger M, Tomas-Loba A, et al. RIF1 is essential for 53BP1-dependent nonhomologous end joining and suppression of DNA double-strand break resection. Mol Cell. 2013;49:858–71.
116. Di Virgilio M, Callen E, Yamane A, Zhang W, Jankovic M, Gitlin AD, et al. Rif1 prevents resection of DNA breaks and promotes immunoglobulin class switching. Science. 2013;339:711–5.

117. Escribano-Díaz C, Orthwein A, Fradet-Turcotte A, Xing M, Young JTF, Tkáč J, et al. A cell cycle-dependent regulatory circuit composed of 53BP1-RIF1 and BRCA1-CtIP controls DNA repair pathway choice. Mol Cell. 2013;49:872–83.
118. Feng L, Fong K-W, Wang J, Wang W, Chen J. RIF1 counteracts BRCA1-mediated end resection during DNA repair. J Biol Chem. 2013;288:11135–43.
119. Zimmermann M, Lottersberger F, Buonomo SB, Sfeir A, De Lange T. 53BP1 regulates DSB repair using Rif1 to control 5′ end resection. Science. 2013;339:700–4.
120. Xu G, Chapman JR, Brandsma I, Yuan J, Mistrik M, Bouwman P, et al. REV7 counteracts DNA double-strand break resection and affects PARP inhibition. Nature. 2015;521:541–4.
121. Tomida J, Takata K, Bhetawal S, Person MD, Chao H, Tang DG, et al. FAM 35A associates with REV 7 and modulates DNA damage responses of normal and BRCA 1-defective cells. EMBO J. 2018;37:e99543.
122. Gupta R, Somyajit K, Narita T, Maskey E, Stanlie A, Kremer M, et al. DNA repair network analysis reveals Shieldin as a key regulator of NHEJ and PARP inhibitor sensitivity. Cell. 2018;173:972–988.e23.
123. Barazas M, Annunziato S, Pettitt SJ, De Krijger I, Ghezraoui H, Roobol SJ, et al. The CST complex mediates end protection at double-strand breaks and promotes PARP inhibitor sensitivity in BRCA1-deficient cells. Cell Rep. 2018;23:2107–18.
124. Isono M, Niimi A, Oike T, Hagiwara Y, Sato H, Sekine R, et al. BRCA1 directs the repair pathway to homologous recombination by promoting 53BP1 Dephosphorylation. Cell Rep. 2017;18:520–32.
125. Densham RM, Morris JR. The BRCA1 Ubiquitin ligase function sets a new trend for remodelling in DNA repair. Nucleus. 2017;8:116–25.
126. Clairmont CS, Sarangi P, Ponnienselvan K, Galli LD, Csete I, Moreau L, et al. TRIP13 regulates DNA repair pathway choice through REV7 conformational change. Nat Cell Biol. 2020;22:87–96.
127. Sarangi P, Clairmont CS, Galli LD, Moreau LA, D'Andrea AD. p31 ^{comet} promotes homologous recombination by inactivating REV7 through the TRIP13 ATPase. Proc Natl Acad Sci. 2020;117:26795–803.
128. Harvey-Jones E, Raghunandan M, Robbez-Masson L, Magraner-Pardo L, Alaguthurai T, Yablonovitch A, et al. Longitudinal profiling identifies co-occurring BRCA1/2 reversions, TP53BP1, RIF1 and PAXIP1 mutations in PARP inhibitor-resistant advanced breast cancer. Ann Oncol. 2024;S0923753424000103
129. Ray Chaudhuri A, Callen E, Ding X, Gogola E, Duarte AA, Lee J-E, et al. Replication fork stability confers chemoresistance in BRCA-deficient cells. Nature. 2016;535:382–7.
130. Cantor SB, Calvo JA. Fork protection and therapy resistance in hereditary breast cancer. Cold Spring Harb Symp Quant Biol. 2017;82:339–48.
131. Quinet A, Lemaçon D, Vindigni A. Replication fork reversal: players and guardians. Mol Cell. 2017;68:830–3.
132. Kolinjivadi AM, Sannino V, De Antoni A, Zadorozhny K, Kilkenny M, Técher H, et al. Smarcal1-mediated fork reversal triggers Mre11-dependent degradation of nascent DNA in the absence of Brca2 and stable Rad51 nucleofilaments. Mol Cell. 2017;67:867–881.e7.
133. Thakar T, Moldovan G-L. The emerging determinants of replication fork stability. Nucleic Acids Res. 2021;49:7224–38.
134. Rondinelli B, Gogola E, Yücel H, Duarte AA, Van De Ven M, Van Der Sluijs R, et al. EZH2 promotes degradation of stalled replication forks by recruiting MUS81 through histone H3 trimethylation. Nat Cell Biol. 2017;19:1371–8.
135. Taglialatela A, Alvarez S, Leuzzi G, Sannino V, Ranjha L, Huang J-W, et al. Restoration of replication fork stability in BRCA1- and BRCA2-deficient cells by inactivation of SNF2-family fork remodelers. Mol Cell. 2017;68:414–430.e8.
136. Dungrawala H, Bhat KP, Le Meur R, Chazin WJ, Ding X, Sharan SK, et al. RADX promotes genome stability and modulates chemosensitivity by regulating RAD51 at replication forks. Mol Cell. 2017;67:374–386.e5.

137. Guillemette S, Serra RW, Peng M, Hayes JA, Konstantinopoulos PA, Green MR, et al. Resistance to therapy in BRCA2 mutant cells due to loss of the nucleosome remodeling factor CHD4. Genes Dev. 2015;29:489–94.
138. Dhoonmoon A, Nicolae CM, Moldovan G-L. The KU-PARP14 axis differentially regulates DNA resection at stalled replication forks by MRE11 and EXO1. Nat Commun. 2022;13:5063.
139. Jackson LM, Dhoonmoon A, Hale A, Dennis KA, Schleicher EM, Nicolae CM, et al. Loss of MED12 activates the TGFβ pathway to promote chemoresistance and replication fork stability in BRCA-deficient cells. Nucleic Acids Res. 2021;49:12855–69.
140. Quinet A, Tirman S, Jackson J, Šviković S, Lemaçon D, Carvajal-Maldonado D, et al. PRIMPOL-mediated adaptive response suppresses replication fork reversal in BRCA-deficient cells. Mol Cell. 2020;77:461–474.e9.
141. Tirman S, Quinet A, Wood M, Meroni A, Cybulla E, Jackson J, et al. Temporally distinct post-replicative repair mechanisms fill PRIMPOL-dependent ssDNA gaps in human cells. Mol Cell. 2021;81:4026–4040.e8.
142. Thakar T, Dhoonmoon A, Straka J, Schleicher EM, Nicolae CM, Moldovan G-L. Lagging strand gap suppression connects BRCA-mediated fork protection to nucleosome assembly through PCNA-dependent CAF-1 recycling. Nat Commun. 2022;13:5323.
143. Hanzlikova H, Kalasova I, Demin AA, Pennicott LE, Cihlarova Z, Caldecott KW. The importance of Poly(ADP-Ribose) polymerase as a sensor of unligated okazaki fragments during DNA replication. Mol Cell. 2018;71:319–331.e3.
144. Maya-Mendoza A, Moudry P, Merchut-Maya JM, Lee M, Strauss R, Bartek J. High speed of fork progression induces DNA replication stress and genomic instability. Nature. 2018;559:279–84.
145. Van Wietmarschen N, Nussenzweig A. Mechanism for synthetic lethality in BRCA-deficient cancers: no longer lagging behind. Mol Cell. 2018;71:877–8.
146. Quinet A, Tirman S, Cybulla E, Meroni A, Vindigni A. To skip or not to skip: choosing repriming to tolerate DNA damage. Mol Cell. 2021;81:649–58.
147. Taglialatela A, Leuzzi G, Sannino V, Cuella-Martin R, Huang J-W, Wu-Baer F, et al. REV1-Polζ maintains the viability of homologous recombination-deficient cancer cells through mutagenic repair of PRIMPOL-dependent ssDNA gaps. Mol Cell. 2021;81:4008–4025.e7.
148. Nusawardhana A, Pale LM, Nicolae CM, Moldovan G-L. USP1-dependent nucleolytic expansion of PRIMPOL-generated nascent DNA strand discontinuities during replication stress. Nucleic Acids Res. 2024;52:2340–54.
149. Hale A, Dhoonmoon A, Straka J, Nicolae CM, Moldovan G-L. Multi-step processing of replication stress-derived nascent strand DNA gaps by MRE11 and EXO1 nucleases. Nat Commun. 2023;14:6265.
150. Rottenberg S, Jaspers JE, Kersbergen A, Van Der Burg E, Nygren AOH, Zander SAL, et al. High sensitivity of BRCA1-deficient mammary tumors to the PARP inhibitor AZD2281 alone and in combination with platinum drugs. Proc Natl Acad Sci. 2008;105:17079–84.
151. Lawlor D, Martin P, Busschots S, Thery J, O'Leary JJ, Hennessy BT, et al. PARP inhibitors as p-glycoprotein substrates. J Pharm Sci. 2014;103:1913–20.
152. Elmeliegy M, Láng I, Smolyarchuk EA, Chung C, Plotka A, Shi H, et al. Evaluation of the effect of P-glycoprotein inhibition and induction on talazoparib disposition in patients with advanced solid tumours. Br J Clin Pharmacol. 2020;86:771–8.
153. Vaidyanathan A, Sawers L, Gannon A-L, Chakravarty P, Scott AL, Bray SE, et al. ABCB1 (MDR1) induction defines a common resistance mechanism in paclitaxel- and olaparib-resistant ovarian cancer cells. Br J Cancer. 2016;115:431–41.
154. Stordal B, Hamon M, McEneaney V, Roche S, Gillet J-P, O'Leary JJ, et al. Resistance to paclitaxel in a cisplatin-resistant ovarian cancer cell line is mediated by P-glycoprotein. Bishop AJR, editor. PLoS One. 2012;7:e40717.

155. Pettitt SJ, Krastev DB, Brandsma I, Dréan A, Song F, Aleksandrov R, et al. Genome-wide and high-density CRISPR-Cas9 screens identify point mutations in PARP1 causing PARP inhibitor resistance. Nat Commun. 2018;9:1849.
156. Du Y, Yamaguchi H, Wei Y, Hsu JL, Wang H-L, Hsu Y-H, et al. Blocking c-Met–mediated PARP1 phosphorylation enhances anti-tumor effects of PARP inhibitors. Nat Med. 2016;22:194–201.
157. Gogola E, Duarte AA, De Ruiter JR, Wiegant WW, Schmid JA, De Bruijn R, et al. Selective loss of PARG restores PARylation and counteracts PARP inhibitor-mediated synthetic lethality. Cancer Cell. 2018;33:1078–1093.e12.
158. Juhász S, Smith R, Schauer T, Spekhardt D, Mamar H, Zentout S, et al. The chromatin remodeler ALC1 underlies resistance to PARP inhibitor treatment. Sci Adv. 2020;6:eabb8626.
159. Verma P, Zhou Y, Cao Z, Deraska PV, Deb M, Arai E, et al. ALC1 links chromatin accessibility to PARP inhibitor response in homologous recombination-deficient cells. Nat Cell Biol. 2021;23:160–71.
160. Hewitt G, Borel V, Segura-Bayona S, Takaki T, Ruis P, Bellelli R, et al. Defective ALC1 nucleosome remodeling confers PARPi sensitization and synthetic lethality with HRD. Mol Cell. 2021;81:767–783.e11.
161. Blessing C, Mandemaker IK, Gonzalez-Leal C, Preisser J, Schomburg A, Ladurner AG. The oncogenic helicase ALC1 regulates PARP inhibitor potency by trapping PARP2 at DNA breaks. Mol Cell. 2020;80:862–875.e6.
162. Murai J, Feng Y, Yu GK, Ru Y, Tang S-W, Shen Y, et al. Resistance to PARP inhibitors by SLFN11 inactivation can be overcome by ATR inhibition. Oncotarget. 2016;7:76534–50.
163. Murai J, Tang S-W, Leo E, Baechler SA, Redon CE, Zhang H, et al. SLFN11 blocks stressed replication forks independently of ATR. Mol Cell. 2018;69:371–384.e6.
164. Sun C, Zhang F, Xiang T, Chen Q, Pandita TK, Huang Y, et al. Phosphorylation of ribosomal protein S6 confers PARP inhibitor resistance in BRCA1-deficient cancers. Oncotarget. 2014;5:3375–85.
165. McCormick A, Donoghue P, Dixon M, O'Sullivan R, O'Donnell RL, Murray J, et al. Ovarian cancers harbor defects in nonhomologous end joining resulting in resistance to rucaparib. Clin Cancer Res. 2017;23:2050–60.
166. Choi YE, Meghani K, Brault M-E, Leclerc L, He YJ, Day TA, et al. Platinum and PARP inhibitor resistance due to overexpression of MicroRNA-622 in BRCA1-mutant ovarian cancer. Cell Rep. 2016;14:429–39.
167. Fukumoto T, Zhu H, Nacarelli T, Karakashev S, Fatkhutdinov N, Wu S, et al. N6-methylation of adenosine of FZD10 mRNA contributes to PARP inhibitor resistance. Cancer Res. 2019;79:2812–20.
168. Soung Y-H, Chung J. Combination treatment strategies to overcome PARP inhibitor resistance. Biomol Ther. 2023;13:1480.
169. Raynaud F, Mina M, Tavernari D, Ciriello G. Pan-cancer inference of intra-tumor heterogeneity reveals associations with different forms of genomic instability. Kool M, editor. PLoS Genet. 2018;14:e1007669.
170. Färkkilä A, Rodríguez A, Oikkonen J, Gulhan DC, Nguyen H, Domínguez J, et al. Heterogeneity and clonal evolution of acquired PARP inhibitor resistance in TP53- and BRCA1 -deficient cells. Cancer Res. 2021;81:2774–87.

Chapter 3
Repair for Estrogen-Induced DNA Damage Requires BRCA1

Kosuke Yamazaki, Kazuto Takayasu, Hisao Masai, and Hiroyuki Sasanuma

Abstract Hereditary breast and ovarian cancer (HBOC) syndrome is a genetic disorder that is diagnosed by the detection of germline mutations in the *BRCA1* or *BRCA2* gene. BRCA1 and BRCA2 are critical in homologous recombination (HR) in conjunction with RAD51 recombinase. BRCA1/2 functions as a tumor suppressor gene, and its loss of function results in chromosomal instability, commonly observed in cancer. In vertebrates, HR is essential for survival, and HR deficiency caused by the mutations in the genes involved in the fundamental processes of HR generally leads to lethality at the cellular level. Since all proliferating cells with hypomorphic mutations in *BRCA1/2* genes, irrespective of their origin, cause HR defects in any proliferating cells, it remains elusive why *BRCA1/2* mutations selectively cause breast and ovarian cancers. This chapter discusses the association between *BRCA1/2* mutations and organ-specific carcinogenesis based on the latest findings on BRCA1 and BRCA2 in DNA repair.

K. Yamazaki (✉) · H. Masai
Genome Dynamics Project, Department of Basic Medical Sciences, Tokyo Metropolitan Institute of Medical Science, Tokyo, Japan

Department of Computational Biology and Medical Sciences, Graduate School of Frontier Sciences, The University of Tokyo, Chiba, Japan
e-mail: yamazaki-ks@igakuken.or.jp

K. Takayasu · H. Sasanuma
Genome Dynamics Project, Department of Basic Medical Sciences, Tokyo Metropolitan Institute of Medical Science, Tokyo, Japan
e-mail: sasanuma-hr@igakuken.or.jp

T. Ohta et al. (eds.), *Practical Guide to Hereditary Breast and Ovarian Cancer III*, https://doi.org/10.1007/978-981-96-6779-6_3

3.1 Introduction

Cell cycle regulation is essential for maintaining genomic stability and for suppressing carcinogenesis. Genomic DNA is constantly under threat from internal and external agents [1]. These potential DNA damages can lead to mutations or cell death if not repaired [2]. Organisms have evolved DNA repair pathways for a wide variety of DNA damages [2]. Ionizing radiation induces double-strand breaks (DSBs), the most dangerous form of DNA damages. DSBs are repaired mainly by homologous recombination (HR) or nonhomologous end joining (NHEJ) pathways [3]. UV- and ROS-induced base lesions are repaired by the nucleotide excision repair (NER) pathway and base lesions by base excision repair (BER), respectively [4].

Interestingly, each pathway functions in a complementary manner, generating a more robust repair system than that generated by more independently operated pathways in response to DNA damage [5–8]. In higher eukaryotes, increased mutation rates lead to carcinogenesis. Genome analyses have revealed numerous mutations in DNA repair genes, such as *BRCA1* and *BRCA2*, in cancer cells, suggesting that DNA damage repair factors function as cancer suppressor genes [9].

Since even a single DSB can be lethal to the cells, DSB must be rapidly recognized and repaired quickly to avoid mutations. DSBs are initially recognized by sensor proteins, followed by transmitting the signal to the mediators and the effector proteins to arrest the cell cycle and repair DSBs. The activities of mediator and effector proteins that function in NHEJ and HR pathways are tightly regulated in a cell-cycle-dependent manner. HR is a repair pathway activated during the S and G_2 phases, while NHEJ can occur throughout the cell cycle [10–12]. The HR pathway is error-free and precisely restores the genomic sequence using a template from the homologous sequences of sister chromatids in close proximity to ensure accurate repair. It is a multistep process and involves more than a hundred proteins. RAD51 recombinase, a homolog of RecA in bacteria, is a central player in HR to catalyze homology search [13, 14]. NHEJ is a predominant pathway for repairing DSBs in vertebrate cells. It also involves a number of proteins, including Ku70, Ku80, DNA-PKcs, XRCC4, and LIG 4 [15, 16]. These proteins recognize and bind to the broken ends of DNA, processing the ends to make them compatible for ligation. The NHEJ pathway is error-prone and causes the loss or gain of nucleotides at the site of the break, leading to mutations or chromosomal rearrangements, potentially generating the cause for cancers. This chapter introduces the role of BRCA1 and BRCA2 in DNA damage repair and would like to discuss why their mutations cause organ-specific carcinogenesis, such as breast and ovarian cancers and prostate cancer.

3.2 BRCA1 and BRCA2 Function in HR and Their Mutations in Cancers

Breast cancer is the second most prevalent cancer in the world and the most common malignancy in women, accounting for more than 10% of all cancers [19]. Mutations of cancer suppressor genes *BRCA1/2* have been isolated as causative genes in hereditary breast and ovarian cancer (HBOC) syndrome. Mutations in *BRCA1* and *BRCA2* are detected in at least 5% of unselected breast cancer patients [20]. Nearly 50% of all HBOC cases can be accounted for by germline mutations in either *BRCA1* or *BRCA2* genes and are associated with early-onset breast and ovarian cancers [21]. It is estimated that approximately 10% of women in the general population will develop breast cancer during their lifetime. In contrast, 40–70% of women who inherit a *BRCA1* or *BRCA2* mutation would develop breast cancer by 80 years of age [22].

FDA has recently approved PARP inhibitors for use in germline *BRCA*-mutated breast cancer [23, 24]. PARP inhibitors are one of the most successful examples of targeted therapy and the first drug for cancer therapy targeting the DNA damage response pathway. Poly (ADP-ribose) polymerase is an enzyme involved in many fundamental cellular processes, including DNA repair, transcription, and differentiation [25–27]. PARP1 and PARP2 enzymes are important in base excision repair, BER [28]. They rapidly associate with SSB sites of genomic DNA and undergo automodification by Poly-ADP ribosylation, a post-translational modification. This, in turn, promotes the dissociation of PARP proteins from SSB sites and stimulates the association of BER repair factors, such as XRCC1, with SSB sites [29]. Although loss or inhibition of PARP1/2 accumulates SSB, these damages can be repaired by alternative pathways, mainly homologous recombination [30]. Unrepaired SSB in *PARP*-deficient cells could be converted into DSBs after the passage of DNA replication forks [31]. The development of PARP inhibitors as anticancer agents is based on the concept of synthetic lethality, where either PARP loss or BRCA deficiency is not lethal, but their combination causes lethality [30]. Thus, *BRCA*-deficient cancer cells are expected to be specifically sensitive to PARP inhibitors.

3.3 The Role of BRCA1 in HR

BRCA1 is a large protein encoding 1863 amino acids in human beings (Fig. 3.1). It has several functional domains, including the RING finger domain and nuclear localization signal (NLS) near its N-terminus and the two BRCT domains near the C-terminus [32]. BRCA1 protein is well known to interact with many other proteins, such as BARD1, ATM, CHEK2, BRIP1, PALB2, RAD51, and TP53. BARD1 forms a

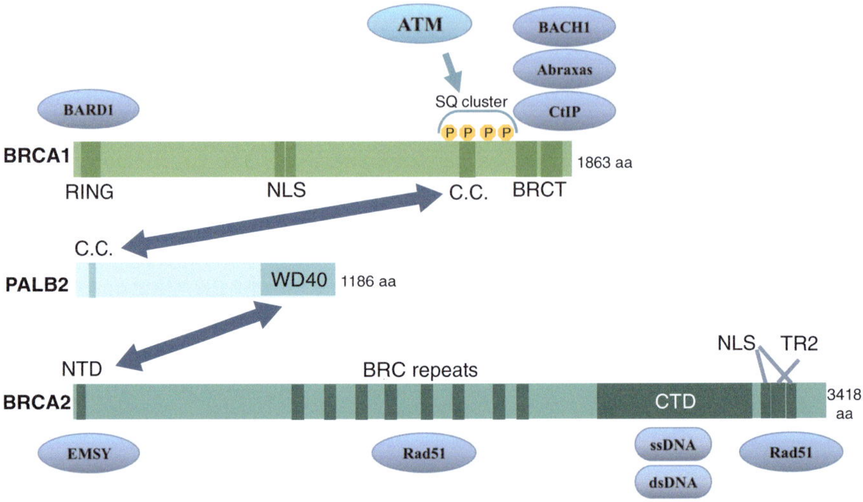

Fig. 3.1 Protein structures of BRCA1, PALB2, and BRCA2. BRCA1 forms a heterodimer with BARD1 via the RING domain. The C-terminus of BRCA1 is important for the interaction with various proteins, such as BATCH1, ABRAXAS, and CtIP. PALB2 mediates the interaction between BRCA1 and BRCA2. The coiled-coil (C.C) domains of both BRCA1 and PALB2 are required for mutual interaction. BRCA2 has eight BRC repeats, which regulate RAD51 dynamics. The C-terminal domain of BRCA2 also has an important role in interaction with RAD51

heterodimer with BRCA1 and functions as a RING-type E3 ubiquitin ligase [32, 33]. The E3 enzymatic activity promotes HR by regulating DSB resection [34]. Recently, biochemical analysis demonstrated that the BRCA1-BARD1 complex facilitates HR via directly interacting with RAD51 recombinase [35]. A coiled-coil repeat of BRCA1 (BRCA1cc) present near the C-terminus, where SQ cluster is also present, is critical for interaction with partner and localizer of BRCA2, PALB2 [36–38]. BRCA1-PALB2 interaction is mediated by a conserved coiled-coil domain (PALB2cc) at the N-terminus of PALB2. PALB2cc is necessary not only for heterodimerization with BRCA1 but also for homodimerization [39, 40]. It would be interesting to investigate how PALB2 could be converted from a homodimer to a heterodimer with BRCA1 when HR is initiated. Interestingly, RNF168, which is involved in the ubiquitination pathway in response to DNA damage, redundantly functions with BRCA1 to promote HR via direct interaction between RNF168 and PALB2 [41, 42].

Two BRCT domains near the C-terminus contribute to diverse biological processes via protein-protein interactions. There are many interacting proteins with the BRCT domains involved not only in DNA repair and cell-cycle checkpoint but also in transcription and chromatin remodeling [32]. Among the interactors, BACH1 and ABRAXAS contribute to DSB repair and G_2-M checkpoint activation [43–45]. The interaction of BRCA1 with CtIP is tightly regulated by CDK-dependent phosphorylation and is critical for DSB resection in HR. [46]

The HR defect caused by BRCA1 loss can be suppressed by the loss of TP53BP1, which is a crucial regulator of nonhomologous end joining (NHEJ) repair [47].

TP53BP1 positively regulates NHEJ-mediated DSB repair by protecting broken ends from DSB resection, a process promoted by BRCA1. During the S/G_2 phases, BRCA1 promotes the removal of TP53BP1 by promoting resection. Loss of BRCA1 does not induce DSB resection, possibly due to the inhibitory effect of TP53BP1 binding on DSB ends. This leads to ligation between inappropriate DNA ends in the S phase. *TP53BP1*$^{-/-}$ cells restore HR and suppress genome instability in *BRCA1*-deficient cells. Interestingly, in mice, deletion of TP53BP1 suppresses embryonic lethality and prevents the chromosomal rearrangements seen in *Brca1*$^{-/-}$ mice. In addition to the above roles, BRCA1 plays important roles in diverse biological reactions, such as meiosis, transcription, apoptosis, and chromosome segregation [48, 49].

3.4 The Role of BRCA1 in the Repair of TOP2-Dependent DNA Damages

We have recently demonstrated that BRCA1 contributes to the repair of topoisomerase 2 (TOP2)-induced DSB in G_1 phase cells [50]. TOP2 is a dimer and a highly conserved enzyme from prokaryotes to mammals [51–53]. TOP2 can resolve topological problems in DNA, including supercoils, knots, and catenanes, frequently occurring during transcription, DNA replication, and chromosome segregation [51, 54]. During catalysis of the TOP2 enzyme, dimerized TOP2 transiently forms a covalent bond with top and bottom DNA strands, leading to TOP2 cleavage complexes (Top2ccs) at the 5′ ends of both DNA strands. After Top2cc formation, the intact DNA duplex passes through the break site of Top2cc, and subsequently, DNA double-strand breaks can be resealed by Top2 itself without activating the DNA damage responses [54]. A recent study reveals in vivo that the catalytic reaction of TOP2 seems erroneous [55]. Failure of Top2 catalysis could lead to the accumulation of Top2-induced double-strand breaks, called abortive Top2ccs. Such abortive Top2ccs are hard to repair, because they inhibit the enzymatic reactions necessary for DSB repair. For instance, in NHEJ, LIG4, an enzyme responsible for ligation, is not able to ligate the DNA ends covalently bound to TOP2. In HR, TOP2ccs at DSB ends block the association of exonucleases responsible for 5′ to 3′ resection necessary for subsequent strand invasion by RAD51. Thus, to repair TOP2-induced DSBs, TOP2 covalently bound to DNA ends should be removed before initiation of DSB repair. Two main pathways have been identified for Top2cc removal (see below).

3.5 TDP2-Dependent Pathway in the Removal of Top2ccs from Genomic DNA

Tyrosyl-DNA phosphodiesterase 2, TDP2, has been identified as the enzyme that explicitly removes TOP2 from the DNA ends [56]. Biochemical analysis has demonstrated that TDP2 can cleave the phosphotyrosine linkage that is formed between tyrosine of the TOP2 catalytic site and the phosphate group of the 5′ DNA end, resulting in the release of TOP2 peptides with tyrosine from the 5′ DNA end [57, 58]. This restores the phosphate group at the 5′ DNA end necessary for ligation by LIG4 in NHEJ. Sumo ligase ZATT facilitates Top2cc removal by enhancing the interaction between TOP2 and TDP2, suggesting a contribution of posttranslational modification to the Top2cc removal [59]. It has been demonstrated that homozygous mutations in TDP2 lacking catalytic activity cause severe neurodegenerative symptoms, such as intellectual disability, epilepsy, and ataxia [60]. Several lines of evidence suggest that TDP2 is required for normal transcription. TDP2 deficiency impairs the induction of androgen-responsive genes in prostate cells and attenuates global transcription in neural cells, indicating a significant contribution of TDP2 to neuronal development and maintenance [60]. In neurons, the repair of abortive Top2ccs that occasionally occur in postmitotic cells requires TDP2 activity for the maintenance of proper transcriptional regulation.

3.6 MRE11-Dependent Pathway

Another pathway is mediated by the MRE11 nuclease, which plays an important role in the DSB recognition and resection of homologous recombination. CtIP, EXOI, MRE11, and DNA2 are all involved in DSB resection [61–63]. While CtIP, EXO1, and DNA2 are all nucleases with the 5′ to 3′ direction, MRE11 nuclease has a 3′ to 5′ exonuclease activity. Since the 3′ overhang is required for invasion into the homologous duplex DNA by RAD51, the direction of MRE11 nuclease is incompatible with the 5′ to 3′ direction of DSB resection. The resolution of this paradox was significantly facilitated by research on meiotic recombination in yeast [64–66]. As initiation of meiotic recombination, DSBs are formed by the conserved SPO11 protein, a topoisomerase 2-like protein. After SPO11 forms a covalent bond with the 5′ end of the DSB, the SPO11 cleavage complex, a complex of SPO11-DNA, can be removed by *MRE11*-dependent endonucleolytic nick of the 5′ strands adjacent to the SPO11 and subsequent MRE11's exonucleolytic digestion DNA strand in the 3′ to 5′direction, i.e., from the nicked site to Spo11-conjugated DSB [65]. CtIP, EXOI, and DNA2 initiate DSB resection from the nick site with the 5′ to 3′ direction for further resection. This repair pathway is considered more versatile not only for removing adducts covalently bound to DNA ends but also for removing proteins tightly associated with DNA ends, such as TP53BP1 and Ku70/80 heterodimers. In the same context as Spo11, Top2ccs have been demonstrated to be removed by Mre11 in yeast and human [55, 67]. *Mre11*-deficient yeast and human cells exhibit hypersensitivity to etoposide, which explicitly inhibits the ligation step of TOP2 catalysis. Interestingly, in humans, loss of MRE11 quickly accumulates Top2cc even in physiological culture conditions, indicating that failure of TOP2 catalysis frequently occurs during the physiological cell cycle. Overexpression of TDP2 partially suppresses cell lethality caused by MRE11 deletion, suggesting a possibility that one of the causes of cell death by MRE11 loss is the Top2cc accumulation [55].

MRE11 in Top2cc removal is active even in the G_1 phase; therefore, its regulation may differ from that in HR.

A recent study reveals that Top2cc removal by MRE11 requires BRCA1 [50]. This requirement is not suppressed by the introduction of TP53BP1 deficiency, indicating that BRCA1's role in Top2cc removal is independent of HR. Loss of BRCA1 abolishes the loading of MRE11 onto Top2ccs, suggesting a regulatory role of BRCA1 in MRE11 recruitment onto Top2cc sites. Further analysis has revealed that the role of UBC13, E2 ubiquitin ligase, contributes to the association of RAP80 and BRCA1 with Top2cc [68]. RAP80 is a member of BRCA1-A complex [17, 18, 69–74], composed of BRCA1, BRCC36, MERIT40, BRCC45, and ABRAXAS. Although the precise role of the BRCA1-A complex remains unclear, RAP80 has unique ubiquitin-interacting motifs (UIMs) to recognize the K63-type ubiquitin chain catalyzed by UBC13 specifically. One possible scenario is that RAP80 links UBC13-RNF8/RNF168-dependent ubiquitin marks on chromatin to proteins necessary for repair by binding to the K63-type ubiquitin chain and subsequent recruitment of the BRCA1 or BRCA-A complex. Loss of UBC13, RAP80, and BRCA1 all exhibit a defect in removing Top2ccs [50]. In sum, in the MRE11-dependent pathway, the UBC13-dependent ubiquitin pathway promotes the removal of Top2cc by recruiting BRCA1-RAP80.

3.7 BRCA1/2 Variants in Cancer

Brca1 and *Brca2* null mice result in early embryonic lethality [75–80]. HR is essential for repairing DNA damage that occurs spontaneously during cell proliferation, and the lethality of *BRCA1/2*-deficient cells is thought to be due to defects in HR. Since HR is essential for all proliferating cells, loss of BRCA1/2 function may result in organ-nonspecific carcinogenesis. However, germline *BRCA1/2* mutations significantly increase the risk of breast and ovarian cancers. Although cells with germline *BRCA1/2* mutations occur in the heterozygous genotype and cancer develops primarily in women, often at a young age, the reason why *BRCA1/2* mutations specifically develop breast and ovarian cancer remains unclear. Currently, over 70,000 *BRCA1/2* variants are registered in the database of BRCA Exchange, and nearly 80% are variants of uncertain significance (VUS) [81]. About 7% of the *BRCA1* and *BRCA2* variants (~4900) in the BRCA Exchange are reviewed by expert panels as pathogenic mutations. More than half of most pathogenic *BRCA1/2* variants are predicted to express truncated proteins due to frameshifts in the coding region by small insertions or deletions. Pathogenic mutations in BRCA1 are predominantly enriched in the N-terminal RING domain and the C-terminal BRCT domains. Saturation mutation analysis regarding the RING and BRCT domains of BRCA1 will enable a more accurate prediction of whether spontaneous VUS, which still exists in large numbers, is pathological or not [82].

3.8 Mice Harboring *BRCA1* Mutations

After discovering BRCA1 and BRCA2, researchers sought to recapitulate the genetic mutations found in cancer patients using mouse models. Many *Brca1* mutant mice have been generated so far. The RING domain mutant mice, *Brca1*$^{I26A/I26A}$ mice, lacking ubiquitin E3 ligase activity, are born at the expected Mendelian ratio and do not show any phenotypes of genome instability, indicating that E3 ligase activity of BRCA1 is dispensable for normal development [83, 84]. In addition, the homozygous mice harboring C61G mutation, one of the most frequently reported missense mutations in the RING domain, exhibit embryonic lethality, and its conditional-mutant mice develop tumors [85]. Since the C61G mutation abolishes not only E3 ligase activity but also BARD1 interaction, while the I26A mutation maintains the BRCA1-BARD1 interaction, BRCA1-BARD1 interaction may be essential for the tumor-suppressive activity of BRCA1. There are some mice lacking the C-terminus segment of BRCA1, which contains two BRCT domains. The C-terminal deletion mice, including homozygous *Brca1*$^{1700T/1700T}$ and *Brca1*$^{5382insC/5382insC}$, all of which could express truncated BRCA1 lacking last BRCT [86], die before embryonic day 10 (E 10) [86, 87], indicating a critical role of BRCT domain in mouse development [88–90]. The homozygous mice lacking a part of the coiled-coil domain near the C-terminus, *Brca1*$^{CC/CC}$ were recently generated [91]. They are born at less than expected Mendelian frequency and show severe defects in development and hematopoiesis, including decreased hematopoietic stem cells, erythrocytes, and leukocytes in peripheral blood [91]. Interestingly, *Brca1*$^{CC/CC}$ MEF cells completely abolish RAD51 loading after IR exposure, most likely due to a lack of PALB2 interaction.

3.9 Estrogen and Breast Cancer

We hypothesized that the association of BRCA mutations with tissue-specific carcinogenesis (breast and ovarian cancers) may be related to the female hormone estrogen (E2). E2 is a lipid-soluble hormone that can penetrate cell membranes. E2 binds to estrogen receptor (ER) localized in the cytoplasm and promotes translocation into the nucleus. The ER in the nucleus acts as a transcription factor to regulate gene expression by binding to *cis*-regulatory elements in promoter and enhancer DNA. E2 strongly facilitates cell proliferation from the G_0/G_1 phase cells by stimulating transcriptional programs necessary for the S-phase, such as MAP kinase, cyclins, and c-myc [92–94]. E2 exposure has also been associated with an increased risk of breast carcinogenesis. It has long been known that high concentrations of E2 in blood are positively correlated with an increased risk of sporadic breast cancer [95, 96]. Recent studies have suggested that hormone-filled therapy, one of the treatments for menopause, raises the incidence of breast cancer [97]. How estrogen is involved in carcinogenesis is unknown, but several lines of evidence suggest that E2 has a genotoxic potential.

3.10 Relationship Between the Repair of Estrogen-Induced Abortive Top2ccs and *BRCA1* Deficiency

Exposure of physiological concentrations (1–10 nM) of E2 to estrogen-receptor-positive human breast cancer epithelial cells MCF7 caused an increasing signal of γH2AX, a DNA damage marker. Cimprich and her colleagues show that estrogen-induced DNA damages are associated with R-loop formation stimulated by estrogen-induced transcription [98]. E2-induced DNA damages are proposed to be caused by the collision of DNA replication forks with the preformed R-loops during the S phase. Our group found that estrogen-induced DNA damages were also observed in the serum-starved G_0/G_1 phase, suggesting that estrogen-induced DNA damages may not be solely due to collisions of DNA replication forks with R-loops [50]. The damages seen in the G_0/G_1 phase depend on TOP2. Loss of TOP2 reduces γH2AX signals, suggesting a contribution of TOP2 catalysis to the induction of DNA damage. Although the significance of these damages in the G_0/G_1 cells remains unknown, TOP2-dependent damages have also been observed in prostate cancer LnCaP cells stimulated by androgen, a male hormone [99, 100]. Interestingly, the breakpoints of oncogenic TMPRSS2-ERG translocation, seen in approximately 50% of patients with prostate cancer [101–103], have been demonstrated to overlap with Top2cc sites. Both TMPRSS2 and ERG genes are androgen-responsive genes, and TOP2 is recruited onto their promoters and enhancers [100]. Unrepaired Top2ccs result in chromosome translocation as an oncogenic driver alternation. In mammary and prostate glands, Top2ccs occasionally accumulate during transcription and DNA replication in response to sex hormones, and unrepaired Top2ccs most likely require TDP2 and/or Mre11 nuclease.

How does TOP2-dependent DNA damage induced by sex hormones affect carcinogenesis in BRCA-deficient cells? Although further analysis is needed to answer the question, as mentioned above, we demonstrated that repairing E2-induced TOP2-mediated DSBs (TOP2-DSBs) also requires BRCA1 (Fig. 3.2). E2 strongly promotes cell proliferation despite abortive Top2cc accumulation (e.g., upregulation of the c-Myc gene). While, in BRCA1-proficient cells, the abortive Top2ccs could be repaired quickly, BRCA1-deficient cells are forced to enter the S-phase from the G_0/G_1 phases in response to E2 despite the presence of a number of unrepaired DNA damages caused by TOP2. Unrepaired Top2ccs would increase chromosome instability, leading to cancer. Interestingly, DNA checkpoint activation that arrests cell cycle progression induced by estrogen does not seem to be observed. Further analysis is needed to investigate whether BRCA2 also contributes to the removal of Top2ccs induced by sex hormones.

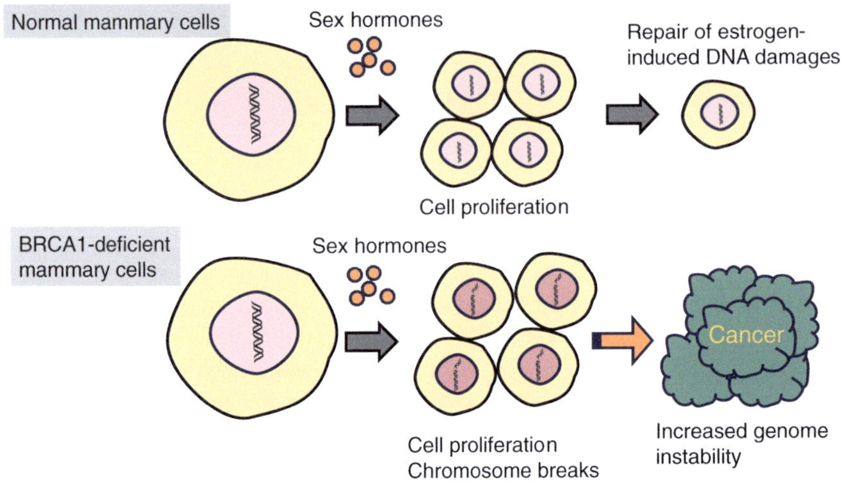

Fig. 3.2 Hypothesis of tumorigenesis caused by BRCA1 mutation. Estrogen strongly promotes cell proliferation. In addition, estrogen also induces DNA damage in mammary epithelial cells, irrespective of the presence/absence of BRCA1. While such DNA damages can be repaired in normal mammary epithelial cells, they are not well repaired in *BRCA1*-deficient cells, resulting in increasing genomic instability that potentially causes cancer

Acknowledgments We thank the members of the Genome Dynamics lab in TMiMS for their helpful comments on the manuscript. This work was supported by the following grants: a Grant-in-Aid from the Ministry of Education, Science, Sport, and Culture to H.S (KAKENHI 19H04267), the Takeda Research Foundation, Astellas Foundation for Research on Metabolic Disorders, Kose Cosmetology research foundation, and Mitsubishi foundation (to H.S.).

References

1. Chatterjee N, Walker GC. Mechanisms of DNA damage, repair, and mutagenesis. Environ Mol Mutagen. 2017;58:235–63.
2. Bauer NC, Corbett AH, Doetsch PW. The current state of eukaryotic DNA base damage and repair. Nucleic Acids Res. 2015;43:10083–101.
3. Seeber A, Gasser SM. Chromatin organization and dynamics in double-strand break repair. Curr Opin Genet Dev. 2017;43:9–16.
4. Fahrer J, Christmann M. DNA alkylation damage by nitrosamines and relevant DNA repair pathways. Int J Mol Sci. 2023;24:4684.
5. Friedberg EC. DNA damage and repair. Nature. 2003;421:436–40.
6. Groelly FJ, Fawkes M, Dagg RA, Blackford AN, Tarsounas M. Targeting DNA damage response pathways in cancer. Nat Rev Cancer. 2023;23:78–94.
7. Pilié PG, Tang C, Mills GB, Yap TA. State-of-the-art strategies for targeting the DNA damage response in cancer. Nat Rev Clin Oncol. 2019;16:81–104.
8. Chitale S, Richly H. Timing of DNA lesion recognition: ubiquitin signaling in the NER pathway. Cell Cycle. 2016;16:163–71.

9. Curtin NJ. DNA repair dysregulation from cancer driver to therapeutic target. Nat Rev Cancer. 2012;12:801–17.
10. Chapman JR, Taylor MRG, Boulton SJ. Playing the end game: DNA double-Strand break repair pathway choice. Mol Cell. 2012;47:497–510.
11. Löbrich M, Jeggo P. A process of resection-dependent nonhomologous end joining involving the goddess Artemis. Trends Biochem Sci. 2017;42:690–701.
12. Kakarougkas A, Jeggo PA. DNA DSB repair pathway choice: an orchestrated handover mechanism. Br J Radiol. 2014;87:20130685.
13. Shinohara A, Ogawa H, Ogawa T. Rad51 protein involved in repair and recombination in S cerevisiae is a RecA-like protein. Cell. 1992;69:457–70.
14. Schwacha A, Kleckner N. Interhomolog bias during meiotic recombination: meiotic functions promote a highly differentiated Interhomolog-only pathway. Cell. 1997;90:1123–35.
15. Waters CA, Strande NT, Wyatt DW, Pryor JM, Ramsden DA. Nonhomologous end joining: a good solution for bad ends. DNA Repair (Amst). 2014;17:39–51.
16. McElhinny SAN, Snowden CM, McCarville J, Ramsden DA. Ku recruits the XRCC4-ligase IV complex to DNA ends. Mol Cell Biol. 2023;20:2996–3003.
17. Wang B, Elledge SJ. Ubc13/Rnf8 ubiquitin ligases control foci formation of the Rap80/Abraxas/Brca1/Brcc36 complex in response to DNA damage. Proc Natl Acad Sci USA. 2007;104:20759–63.
18. Yan J, et al. The ubiquitin-interacting motif-containing protein RAP80 interacts with BRCA1 and functions in DNA damage repair response. Cancer Res. 2007;67:6647–56.
19. Simon A, Robb K. Breast cancer. In: Cambridge handbook of psychology, health and medicine, Second Edition; 2022. p. 577–80.
20. Trainer AH, et al. The role of BRCA mutation testing in determining breast cancer therapy. Nat Rev Clin Oncol. 2010;7:708–17.
21. Genetics of Breast and Gynecologic Cancers (PDQ®) – NCI.
22. Narod SA. BRCA mutations in the management of breast cancer: the state of the art. Nat Rev Clin Oncol. 2010;7:702–7.
23. Baselga J, et al. A positive defect. Nat Rev Cancer. 2005;5:333.
24. Bryant HE, et al. Specific killing of BRCA2-deficient tumours with inhibitors of poly(ADP-ribose) polymerase. Nature. 2005;434:913–7.
25. Chaitanya GV, Alexander JS, Babu PP. PARP-1 cleavage fragments: signatures of cell-death proteases in neurodegeneration. Cell Commun Signal. 2010;8:1–11.
26. Zong W, Gong Y, Sun W, Li T, Wang ZQ. PARP1: liaison of chromatin remodeling and transcription. Cancers. 2022;14:4162.
27. Pazzaglia S, Pioli C. Multifaceted role of PARP-1 in DNA repair and inflammation: pathological and therapeutic implications in cancer and non-cancer diseases. Cells. 2019;9:41.
28. Caldecott KW. Mammalian DNA base excision repair: dancing in the moonlight. DNA Repair (Amst). 2020;93:102921.
29. Hegde ML, Hazra TK, Mitra S. Early steps in the DNA base excision/single-strand interruption repair pathway in mammalian cells. Cell Res. 2008;18:27–47.
30. Tung NM, Garber JE. BRCA1/2 testing: therapeutic implications for breast cancer management. Br J Cancer. 2018;119:141–52.
31. Bhamidipati D, Haro-Silerio JI, Yap TA, Ngoi N. PARP inhibitors: enhancing efficacy through rational combinations. Br J Cancer. 2023;1–13:904.
32. Narod SA, Foulkes WD. BRCA1 and BRCA2: 1994 and beyond. Nat Rev Cancer. 2004;4:665–76.
33. Roy R, Chun J, Powell SN. BRCA1 and BRCA2: different roles in a common pathway of genome protection. Nat Rev Cancer. 2011;12:68–78.
34. Densham RM, et al. Human BRCA1–BARD1 ubiquitin ligase activity counteracts chromatin barriers to DNA resection. Nat Struct Mol Biol. 2016;23:647–55.

35. Tarsounas M, Sung P. The antitumorigenic roles of BRCA1–BARD1 in DNA repair and replication. Nat Rev Mol Cell Biol. 2020;21:284–99.
36. Zhang F, Fan Q, Ren K, Andreassen PR. PALB2 functionally connects the breast cancer susceptibility proteins BRCA1 and BRCA2. Mol Cancer Res. 2009;7:1110–8.
37. Sy SMH, Huen MSY, Chen J. PALB2 is an integral component of the BRCA complex required for homologous recombination repair. Proc Natl Acad Sci USA. 2009;106:7155–60.
38. Zhang F, et al. PALB2 links BRCA1 and BRCA2 in the DNA-damage response. Curr Biol. 2009;19:524–9.
39. Sy SMH, Huen MSY, Zhu Y, Chen J. PALB2 regulates Recombinational repair through chromatin association and Oligomerization. J Biol Chem. 2009;284:18302–10.
40. Buisson R, Masson JY. PALB2 self-interaction controls homologous recombination. Nucleic Acids Res. 2012;40:10312–23.
41. Luijsterburg, M. S. *et al.* A PALB2-interacting domain in RNF168 couples homologous recombination to DNA break-induced chromatin ubiquitylation. elife. 2017;6.
42. Zong D, et al. BRCA1 Haploinsufficiency is masked by RNF168-mediated chromatin Ubiquitylation. Mol Cell. 2019;73:1267–1281.e7.
43. Cantor SB, et al. BACH1, a novel helicase-like protein, interacts directly with BRCA1 and contributes to its DNA repair function. Cell. 2001;105:149–60.
44. Yu X, Chini CCS, He M, Mer G, Chen J. The BRCT domain is a Phospho-protein binding domain. Science. 2003;1979(302):639–42.
45. Wang B, et al. Abraxas and RAP80 form a BRCA1 protein complex required for the DNA damage response. Science. 2007;1979(316):1194–8.
46. Yun MH, Hiom K. CtIP-BRCA1 modulates the choice of DNA double-strand-break repair pathway throughout the cell cycle. Nature. 2009;459:460–3.
47. Bunting SF, et al. 53BP1 inhibits homologous recombination in Brca1-deficient cells by blocking resection of DNA breaks. Cell. 2010;141:243–54.
48. Xu X, et al. Genetic interactions between tumor suppressors Brca1 and p53 in apoptosis, cell cycle and tumorigenesis. Nat Genet. 2001;28:266–71.
49. Matsuzawa A, et al. The BRCA1/BARD1-interacting protein OLA1 functions in centrosome regulation. Mol Cell. 2014;53:101–14.
50. Sasanuma H, et al. BRCA1 ensures genome integrity by eliminating estrogen-induced pathological topoisomerase II-DNA complexes. Proc Natl Acad Sci USA. 2018;115:E10642–51.
51. Pommier Y, Sun Y, Huang SYN, Nitiss JL. Roles of eukaryotic topoisomerases in transcription, replication and genomic stability. Nat Rev Mol Cell Biol. 2016;17:703–21.
52. Pommier Y. Drugging topoisomerases: lessons and challenges. ACS Chem Biol. 2013;8:82–95.
53. Ashour ME, Atteya R, El-Khamisy SF. Topoisomerase-mediated chromosomal break repair: an emerging player in many games. Nat Rev Cancer. 2015;15:137–51.
54. Uusküla-Reimand L, Wilson MD. Untangling the roles of TOP2A and TOP2B in transcription and cancer. Sci Adv. 2022;8:eadd4920.
55. Hoa NN, et al. Mre11 is essential for the removal of lethal topoisomerase 2 covalent cleavage complexes. Mol Cell. 2016;64:580–92.
56. Ledesma FC, El Khamisy SF, Zuma MC, Osborn K, Caldecott KW. A human 5′-tyrosyl DNA phosphodiesterase that repairs topoisomerase-mediated DNA damage. Nature. 2009;461:674–8.
57. Zeng Z, Cortés-Ledesma F, El Khamisy SF, Caldecott KW. TDP2/TTRAP is the major 5′-Tyrosyl DNA phosphodiesterase activity in vertebrate cells and is critical for cellular resistance to topoisomerase II-induced DNA damage. J Biol Chem. 2011;286:403–9.
58. Pommier Y, et al. Tyrosyl-DNA-phosphodiesterases (TDP1 and TDP2). DNA Repair (Amst). 2014;19:114–29.
59. Schellenberg MJ, et al. ZATT (ZNF451)–mediated resolution of topoisomerase 2 DNA-protein cross-links. Science. 2017;1979(357):1412–6.
60. Gómez-Herreros F, et al. TDP2 protects transcription from abortive topoisomerase activity and is required for normal neural function. Nat Genet. 2014;46:516–21.

61. Hoa NN, et al. Relative contribution of four nucleases, CtIP, Dna2, Exo1 and Mre11, to the initial step of DNA double-strand break repair by homologous recombination in both the chicken DT40 and human TK6 cell lines. Genes Cells. 2015;20:1059–76.
62. Mimitou EP, Symington LS. DNA end resection: many nucleases make light work. DNA Repair (Amst). 2009;8:983–95.
63. Mimitou EP, Symington LS. DNA end resection—unraveling the tail. DNA Repair (Amst). 2011;10:344–8.
64. Neale MJ, Pan J, Keeney S. Endonucleolytic processing of covalent protein-linked DNA double-strand breaks. Nature. 2005;436:1053–7.
65. Garcia V, Phelps SEL, Gray S, Neale MJ. Bidirectional resection of DNA double-strand breaks by Mre11 and Exo1. Nature. 2011;479:241–4.
66. Daley JM, Niu H, Miller AS, Sung P. Biochemical mechanism of DSB end resection and its regulation. DNA Repair (Amst). 2015;32:66–74.
67. Hartsuiker E, Neale MJ, Carr AM. Distinct requirements for the Rad32Mre11 nuclease and Ctp1CtIP in the removal of covalently bound topoisomerase I and II from DNA. Mol Cell. 2009;33:117–23.
68. Akagawa R, et al. UBC13-mediated ubiquitin signaling promotes removal of blocking adducts from DNA double-Strand breaks. iScience. 2020;23:101027.
69. Kim H, Huang J, Chen J. CCDC98 is a BRCA1-BRCT domain–binding protein involved in the DNA damage response. Nat Struct Mol Biol. 2007;14:710–5.
70. Wang B, Hurov K, Hofmann K, Elledge SJ. NBA1, a new player in the Brca1 A complex, is required for DNA damage resistance and checkpoint control. Genes Dev. 2009;23:729–39.
71. Shao G, et al. MERIT40 controls BRCA1-Rap80 complex integrity and recruitment to DNA double-strand breaks. Genes Dev. 2009;23:740–54.
72. Feng L, Huang T, Chen J. MERIT40 facilitates BRCA1 localization and DNA damage repair. Genes Dev. 2009;23:719–28.
73. Liu Z, Wu J, Yu X. CCDC98 targets BRCA1 to DNA damage sites. Nat Struct Mol Biol. 2007;14:716–20.
74. Kim H, Chen J, Yu X. Ubiquitin-binding protein RAP80 mediates BRCA1-dependent DNA damage response. Science. 2007;1979(316):1202–5.
75. Hakem R, et al. The tumor suppressor gene Brca1 is required for embryonic cellular proliferation in the mouse. Cell. 1996;85:1009–23.
76. Liu CY, Flesken-Nikitin A, Li S, Zeng Y, Lee WH. Inactivation of the mouse Brca1 gene leads to failure in the morphogenesis of the egg cylinder in early postimplantation development. Genes Dev. 1996;10:1835–43.
77. Gowen LC, Johnson BL, Latour AM, Sulik KK, Koller BH. Brca1 deficiency results in early embryonic lethality characterized by neuroepithelial abnormalities. Nat Genet. 1996;12:191–4.
78. Shen SX, et al. A targeted disruption of the murine Brca1 gene causes gamma-irradiation hypersensitivity and genetic instability. Oncogene. 1998;17:3115–24.
79. Michelle Bennett L, et al. Brca2-null embryonic survival is prolonged on the BALB/c genetic background. Mol Carcinog. 2000;28:174–83.
80. Ludwig T, Chapman DL, Papaioannou VE, Efstratiadis A. Targeted mutations of breast cancer susceptibility gene homologs in mice: lethal phenotypes of Brca1, Brca2, Brca1/Brca2, Brca1/p53, and Brca2/p53 nullizygous embryos. Genes Dev. 1997;11:1226–41.
81. BRCA Exchange. https://brcaexchange.org/.
82. Findlay GM, et al. Accurate classification of BRCA1 variants with saturation genome editing. Nature. 2018;562:217–22.
83. Reid LJ, et al. E3 ligase activity of BRCA1 is not essential for mammalian cell viability or homology-directed repair of double-strand DNA breaks. Proc Natl Acad Sci USA. 2008;105:20876–81.
84. Shakya R, et al. BRCA1 tumor suppression depends on BRCT phosphoprotein binding, but not its E3 ligase activity. Science. 2011;1979(334):525–8.

85. Drost R, et al. BRCA1 RING function is essential for tumor suppression but dispensable for therapy resistance. Cancer Cell. 2011;20:797–809.
86. Hohenstein P, et al. A targeted mouse Brca1 mutation removing the last BRCT repeat results in apoptosis and embryonic lethality at the headfold stage. Oncogene. 2001;20:2544–50.
87. Nacson J, et al. BRCA1 mutation-specific responses to 53BP1 loss-induced homologous recombination and PARP inhibitor resistance. Cell Rep. 2018;24:3513–3527.e7.
88. Mgbemena VE, et al. Distinct Brca1 mutations differentially reduce hematopoietic stem cell function. Cell Rep. 2017;18:947–60.
89. Liang Y, et al. Structural analysis of BRCA1 reveals modification hotspot. Sci Adv. 2017;3:e1701386.
90. Metcalfe KA, et al. Screening for founder mutations in BRCA1 and BRCA2 in unselected Jewish women. J Clin Oncol. 2010;28:387–91.
91. Nacson J, et al. BRCA1 mutational complementation induces synthetic viability. Mol Cell. 2020;78:951–959.e6.
92. Chakravarty D, et al. Extranuclear functions of ER impact invasive migration and metastasis by breast cancer cells. Cancer Res. 2010;70:4092–101.
93. Zheng S, et al. 17β-estradiol enhances breast cancer cell motility and invasion via extra-nuclear activation of actin-binding protein Ezrin. PLoS One. 2011;6:e22439.
94. Yamaga R, et al. RNA sequencing of MCF-7 breast cancer cells identifies novel estrogen-responsive genes with functional estrogen receptor-binding sites in the vicinity of their transcription start sites. Horm Cancer. 2013;4:222–32.
95. Colditz GA. Relationship between estrogen levels, use of hormone replacement therapy, and breast cancer. J Natl Cancer Inst. 1998;90:814–23.
96. Ark M, Lemons C, Aul P, Oss G. Estrogen and the risk of breast cancer. N Engl J Med. 2001;344:276–85.
97. Shah NR, Borenstein J, Dubois RW. Postmenopausal hormone therapy and breast cancer: a systematic review and meta-analysis. Menopause. 2005;12:668–78.
98. Stork CT, et al. Co-transcriptional R-loops are the main cause of estrogen-induced DNA damage. elife. 2016;5
99. Al Mahmud MR, et al. TDP2 suppresses genomic instability induced by androgens in the epithelial cells of prostate glands. Genes Cells. 2020;25:450–65.
100. Haffner MC, et al. Androgen-induced TOP2B-mediated double-strand breaks and prostate cancer gene rearrangements. Nat Genet. 2010;42:668–75.
101. Hermans KG, et al. TMPRSS2:ERG fusion by translocation or interstitial deletion is highly relevant in androgen-dependent prostate cancer, but is bypassed in late-stage androgen receptor-negative prostate cancer. Cancer Res. 2006;66:10658–63.
102. Clark J, et al. Diversity of TMPRSS2-ERG fusion transcripts in the human prostate. Oncogene. 2006;26:2667–73.
103. Perner S, et al. TMPRSS2:ERG fusion-associated deletions provide insight into the heterogeneity of prostate cancer. Cancer Res. 2006;66:8337–41.

Part II
Breast

Chapter 4
Radiation Sensitivity for *BRCA* Mutation Carriers

Reiko Yoshida

Abstract Radiation is widely used in medical imaging diagnosis and irradiation therapy, leveraging its penetrating and ionizing capabilities. It has also proven beneficial in cancer treatment. However, the risk of cancer development due to radiation-induced cellular damage is recognized as a stochastic effect. Consequently, radiation is administered with care in medical settings, especially in cases involving hereditary diseases where repairing cell damage poses significant challenges. *BRCA1/2* genes exhibit high penetrance in breast, ovarian, prostate, and pancreatic cancers, known for promoting tumors through autosomal dominant inheritance, adult-onset, multiple cancer types, and deficiencies in homologous recombination repair. Concerning breast-conserving surgery with radiation and radiation exposure during imaging and potential secondary cancer risks, the stochastic effects of radiation on individuals carrying germline *BRCA1/2* mutations in a single-allele remain inconclusive. Therefore, it is important to continue accumulating and accurately interpreting evidence to determine appropriate risk management methods for each patient based on the cancer susceptibility of *BRCA1/2* mutation carriers. This process should consider medical evidence, the patient's age, cosmetic appearance, cost-effectiveness, and patient's satisfaction.

Keywords *BRCA1* · *BRCA2* · Radiation sensitivity · DNA damage · DNA repair · Homologous recombination · Breast-conserving

---

R. Yoshida (✉)
Saitama Cancer Center, Department of Medical Genetics and Genomics, Saitama, Japan
e-mail: yoshida.reiko@saitama-pho.co.jp

T. Ohta et al. (eds.), *Practical Guide to Hereditary Breast and Ovarian Cancer III*, https://doi.org/10.1007/978-981-96-6779-6_4

4.1 Introduction

Breast cancer is the most common cancer among women in developed countries [1]. Risk factors for developing breast cancer generally include environmental factors such as obesity, few pregnancies and childbirths, and prolonged exposure to estrogen; however, it is also known that some individuals have genetic predispositions to cancer. Genes associated with hereditary cancer syndromes are tumor suppressors that produce proteins involved in DNA repair pathways of external and internal damage. This chapter discusses the current consensus on medical management based on biological and clinical knowledge regarding the effects of radiation exposure, an external factor of cell damage, *BRCA1/2* carriers, and other representative genes for hereditary breast and ovarian cancer syndromes.

4.2 Radiation Used in Medicine

Radiation exists in nature, such as in food, earth, and space, but the radiation used in medicine is artificially produced using radiation generators and accelerators. The important properties of radiation in medicine include penetration and ionization. Two types of radiation exist: electromagnetic waves (radio waves and light) and particle beams. Electromagnetic waves exhibit wave properties, and as their wavelength shortens, they progress from radio waves to light, then to ultraviolet rays, and finally to higher-energy forms of radiation (X-rays and γ- rays). Particle beams, meanwhile, constitute a form of radiation (α- particles, β-particles, etc.) composed of particles such as electrons, protons, and neutrons, which are fundamental components of atoms constituting all substances. Radiation can be generated by the collision of electrons accelerated by a high voltage to generate X-rays or accelerating particles. Alternatively, radiation from radioisotopes (RI) can also be used. When an RI atom transits from an unstable to a stable state, it emits electromagnetic waves (γ-rays), electrons (β-particles), and helium nuclei composed of two protons and two neutrons (α-particles) [2, 3].

4.3 Penetration and Ionization

The penetration power varies depending on the type of radiation used. α-particles and β-particles have lower penetrating power compared to X-rays and γ-rays. X-rays and γ-rays can penetrate materials like paper, thin metals such as aluminum, and human tissues but are stopped by lead. Contrastingly, particle beams vary in penetrating power based on their energy. In particle beam therapy, adjusting the energy allows beams to penetrate the body's surface and target the cancerous area effectively.

This process, in which radiation directly affects biological molecules, is called direct action. Ionization occurs when radiation transfers its energy to the atoms and molecules within a substance, causing electrons to be separated from their respective atoms and molecules. This process of ionization damages DNA (genes) when radiation passes through human cells. Cancer cells, which proliferate actively, are particularly vulnerable to ionization, because their DNA repair mechanisms may not function effectively, leading to cell death or impairment of growth. Human cells are made up of approximately 70% water; thus, water ionization is more likely to occur. This ionization produces radicals, chemically reactive components that damage living organisms. This process is called an indirect action. Considering these properties, radiation is used in medicine for diagnostic imaging (e.g., X-rays and CT scans) and radiation therapy (e.g., external beam radiation and sealed brachytherapy) [4].

4.4 Radiation and Cell Damage

DNA is a molecule composed of many nucleotides, each consisting of a sugar, base, and phosphate. The four bases, adenine, guanine, cytosine, and thymine, form a double-stranded structure by pairing with each other through hydrogen bonds, forming a double-helical structure. Cells are exposed to exogenous and endogenous stressors that cause various types of DNA damage, including base damage, base loss, and DNA strand breaks [5].

Base damage: A molecule undergoes a chemical change due to the oxidation of the base or breaking of a double bond. More than 100 types of base damages were observed.

Base loss: The chemical bonds between the base and sugar are broken, causing the base to be lost.

DNA strand breaks: Sugars and phosphates that constitute the backbone of the DNA strand are damaged and cause the DNA strand to break. Single- and double-stranded DNA breaks exist.

For example, 1 Gy of X-ray radiation causes hundreds of base damage, about a thousand DNA single-strand breaks, and approximately 40 double-strand breaks per cell [6]. DNA damage induces the DNA damage response and activates several DNA repair pathways. If such damage is not properly repaired, mutations occur, and genomic instability spreads, which is one of the characteristics of cancer that promotes tumors. Proliferating cancer cells are mutagenic and lack functional DNA repair pathways, making them susceptible to DNA damage. The primary repair mechanisms involved in radiation-induced DDR include base excision repair, DNA double-stranded break repair, and checkpoint mechanisms [7].

Base excision repair (BER): In humans, radiation-induced damages, such as base damage, base loss, and DNA single-strand breaks, are repaired by a common pathway called base excision repair. DNA repair is achieved by recognizing damaged bases in the DNA, cleaving the damaged bases, and filling gaps based on information from the template strand. Enzymes, such as DNA glycosylase, AP endonuclease, DNA polymerase, and DNA ligase, are involved in these reactions [8].

DNA double-strand break repair: When double-stranded DNA breaks, it cannot be repaired using the complementary strand of DNA as a template, as in BER; therefore, the repair pathway is complex and requires many proteins. In humans, double-stranded DNA breaks prevent cell division, ultimately leading to chromosomal abnormalities and cell death. The effects of radiation on living organisms largely depend on the frequency of double-stranded DNA breaks and their repair efficiency. There are two types of DNA double-stranded break repair pathways. One is the non-homologous end joining (NHEJ) pathway, in which DNA ligase removes the damaged site at the end and rejoins. NHEJ is a repair pathway prone to mutations, because several to several dozen bases are often missing from the cut end of DNA during the repair process. The second mechanism is homologous recombination repair (HRR). This repair method uses chromosomes (sister chromatids) that have the same genetic information formed after DNA replication as a template and is limited to the latter half of the S phase to the G2 phase of the cell cycle, when sister chromatids exist. One of the DNA strands at the cut DNA end was degraded to expose the single-stranded DNA. Then, the DNA of the homologous sequence of the undamaged sister chromatid was cleaved, allowing the previously exposed single-stranded DNA to slide in and form base pairs. After exchanging DNA strands in this manner, the damaged site is perfectly repaired by DNA polymerase, using the DNA strand of the undamaged sister chromatid as a template [7, 9]. BRCA1 and BRCA2 function in these HRR mechanisms.

Checkpoint mechanism: Besides the DNA damage repair mechanism, eukaryotic cells are equipped with a checkpoint mechanism that protects the body from DNA damage. The checkpoint mechanism monitors DNA abnormalities in the nucleus; if damage occurs, it stops cell proliferation or induces cell death (apoptosis). It is a signaling pathway consisting of many proteins, with ATM at the top. ATM is a DNA repair enzyme that promotes repair reactions by enhancing the activity of several DNA repair enzymes. ATM also activates proteins that stop cell cycle progression and cell proliferation until the repair reaction is completed. This prevents cells from dividing and proliferating while leaving DNA damaged, which could lead to incorrect genetic information being passed on to the next generation, causing mutations or chromosomal abnormalities. If the amount of DNA damage exceeds the repair capacity of the cell, ATM activates multiple proteins, including p53, and actively induces cell death [10].

4.5 Radiation Exposure and Its Effects on Humans

Radiation exposure damages cellular DNA through direct and indirect effects. When the radiation dose is small, most of the damage can be repaired by cellular mechanisms. However, high doses of radiation overwhelm these repair processes, leading to insufficient repair and potential health effects on the human body. This phenomenon is known as the deterministic effect, which exhibits a threshold specific to each organ. For deterministic effects, the threshold dose is the level at which symptoms appear in 1% of individuals exposed to the same dose; certain conditions like hair loss, cataracts, and skin disorders may manifest above this threshold. Contrastingly, for cancer induction, no specific threshold dose exists below which there is no risk. Factors like smoking and alcohol consumption can magnify the carcinogenic effects of radiation, making it impossible to establish a clear threshold. Cancer risk from radiation exposure is considered a stochastic effect, where the likelihood of developing cancer increases with radiation exposure dose. Unlike deterministic effects, stochastic effects do not have a threshold dose; instead, they are evaluated based on the relative risk of cancer development.

Ethical constraints prevent prospective clinical studies on long-term radiation exposure effects, necessitating reliance on epidemiological studies from incidents like wars or accidents involving sudden radiation exposure to estimate cancer risks in humans [11]. The risk of cancer varies depending on the organ affected and the age at the time of exposure. While deterministic effects occur when exceeding a threshold dose, the stochastic effect poses a continuous risk of cancer development due to radiation exposure. Some genetic diseases with germline mutations in genes that belong to the DNA repair or checkpoint pathways have various phenotypes, such as high cancer incidence, immunodeficiency, neurological symptoms, and premature aging. Accumulation of DNA damage is generally associated with cancer and degenerative diseases, and many of these phenotypes affect specific cells and organs. In autosomal recessive genetic diseases, one or more DNA repair proteins are lost in all cells, impairing DNA damage repair. For example, Fanconi anemia may be affected by several proteins involved in homologous recombination (HR), and its symptoms include developmental abnormalities and bone marrow failure [12]. Ataxia-telangiectasia is caused by loss of function due to biallelic mutations in *ATM* and is associated with movement disorders, growth retardation, immunodeficiency, and a high risk of developing cancer [13]. Currently, the American Society for Radiation Oncology (ASTRO) guidelines list the following hereditary diseases that are clinically and cellularly radiosensitive to cancer development: autosomal recessive ataxia-telangiectasia (*ATM*), autosomal recessive/X-linked recessive Fanconi anemia (*FANCA-FANCW*), autosomal dominant Gorlin syndrome (*PTCH1*), Li-Fraumeni syndrome (*TP53*), and retinoblastoma (*RB1*), which are associated with exposure to radiation therapy for malignant tumors in childhood [14]. *BRCA1* and *BRCA2* are autosomal dominant, and carriers have an increased risk of breast, ovarian, prostate, and pancreatic cancers. The function of BRCA is lost in tumor cells, while normal cells typically retain heterozygosity. Therefore, normal cells are not necessarily expected to respond differently to radiation than *BRCA1/2* wild-type cells [14]. Moreover, only 15% of DNA double-stranded breaks are repaired via homologous recombination (HR). Tumor cells with a single *BRCA1* or *BRCA2* allele do not exhibit genomic signatures associated with HR deficiency [14–16]. According to ASTRO guidelines, *BRCA1/2* carriers are not classified as radiosensitive.

4.6 Approach to Radiation Exposure in Medicine for BRCA1/2 Mutation Carriers

Multiple clinical guidelines have been established for *BRCA1/2* mutation carriers. Global guidelines for breast-conserving surgery with radiation and breast surveillance with radiation exposure have been presented (Tables 4.1 and 4.2) [17–22].

4.6.1 *Breast-Conserving Surgery for* BRCA1/2 *Mutation Carriers*

In the past, there was strong concern about increased secondary cancers due to radiation sensitivity in *BRCA1/2* mutation carriers, and breast-conserving surgery with radiation was generally avoided. In recent years, many studies have been unable to demonstrate an association between radiation exposure and increased cancer risk owing to a lack of consistency in the results of clinical studies, long-term follow-ups, adjustment of background factors, and systematic reviews with appropriate comparison subjects and outcome settings. The results of the systematic review of the Japanese HBOC guidelines [23] are shown in Fig. 4.1. A meta-analysis was conducted on 13 cohort studies [24–36]. In *BRCA1/2* mutation carriers, the risk of ipsilateral breast tumor recurrence (IBTR) following breast-conserving surgery is

Table 4.1 Guidelines for breast-conserving surgery with radiation in *BRCA* mutation carriers

Guideline	Content
NCCN Breast 2024 ver3 [17]	BCS is contraindicated for patients with homozygous (biallelic) inactivation for ATM mutation Relative contraindications to lumpectomy include those with a known or suspected genetic predisposition to breast cancer who may have an increased risk of ipsilateral breast recurrence or contralateral breast cancer with BCT or who may be considered for prophylactic bilateral mastectomy for risk reduction as per the criteria in the NCCN Guidelines for genetic/familial high-risk assessment: Breast, ovarian, and pancreatic cancers or may have known or suspected li-Fraumeni syndrome
ASCO [18]	Germline BRCA status should not preclude a patient with newly diagnosed breast cancer otherwise eligible for breast-conserving therapy (BCT) from receiving BCT (type: Formal consensus; evidence quality: Intermediate; strength of recommendation: Moderate)
ESMO [19]	In women with stage I-III high-risk PV-associated breast cancer (not including TP53), breast conservation with therapeutic radiation is a safe alternative to RRM
ASBrS [20]	Radiation is relatively contraindicated in patients with TP53 pathogenic variants (associated with li-Fraumeni syndrome) due to their increased risk of developing radiation-induced secondary malignancies

Table 4.2 Guidelines for breast surveillance, including diagnostic radiology, in *BRCA* mutation carriers

Guideline	Content
NCCN Genetic/Familial High-Risk Assessment: Breast, Ovarian, and Pancreatic 2024 ver3 [21]	Breast awareness starts at the age of 18 years Clinical breast exam every 6–12 months, starting at age 25 years Breast screening: Age 25–29 years, annual breast MRI screening with and without contrast (or mammogram, only if MRI is unavailable) or individualized based on family history if a breast cancer diagnosis before age 30 is present. Age 30–75 years, annual mammogram and breast MRI screening with and without contrast. Age >75 years, management should be considered on an individual basis
ESMO [19]	*BRCA1* carriers Intensified surveillance with MRI from age 30 or 5 years younger than the youngest family member with breast cancer Imaging should be carried out at 6-month intervals If MRI was not available for a 6-month screening, consider the following options: in carriers 30–39 years of age, US with/without mammography in carriers ≧40 years of age, mammography with/without US *BRCA2* carriers Intensified surveillance with MRI from age 30 or 5 years younger than the youngest family member with breast cancer Imaging should be performed annually
NICE [22]	Offer annual mammographic surveillance to women: Aged 40 to 69 years with a known BRCA1 or BRCA2 mutation Offer mammographic surveillance as part of the population screening program for women Aged 70 years and over with a known BRCA1 or BRCA2 mutation Offer annual MRI surveillance to women: Aged 30 to 49 years with a known BRCA1 or BRCA2 mutation Do not offer MRI to women: Aged 50 to 69 years with a known BRCA1 or BRCA2 mutation unless mammography has shown a dense breast pattern Aged 20 to 29 years with a known BRCA1 or BRCA2 mutation Consider annual mammographic surveillance for women: Aged 30 to 39 years with a known BRCA1 or BRCA2 mutation Do not routinely offer ultrasound surveillance to women at moderate risk or high risk of breast cancer, but consider it When MRI surveillance would normally be offered but is not suitable (e.g., because of claustrophobia.) When results of mammography or MRI are difficult to interpret

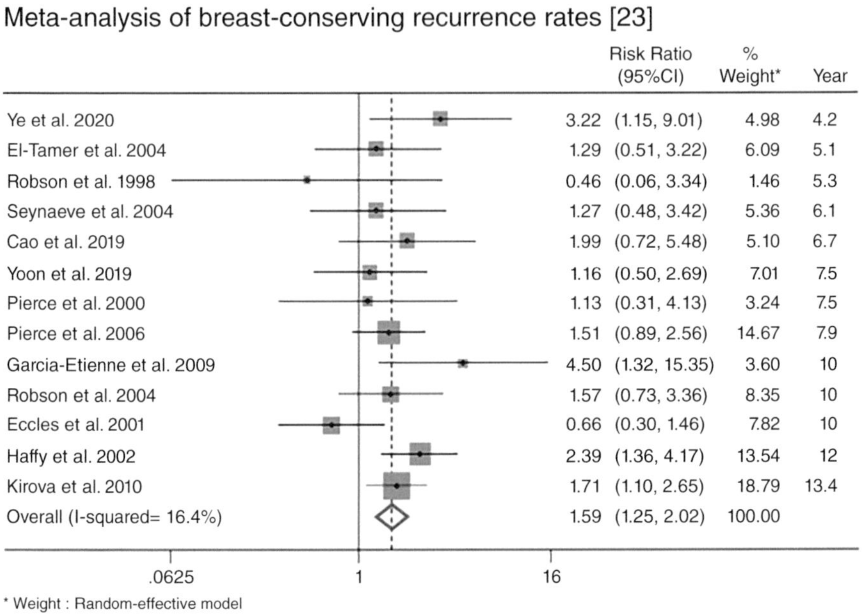

Fig. 4.1 Meta-analysis of breast-conserving recurrence rates [23] (*Weight:Random-effective model)

significantly higher compared to patients with sporadic breast cancer (RR: 1.589, 95% CI: 1.247–2.024). Moreover, in analyses spanning seven years or more, the RR was 1.505 (1.184–1.913), and for ten years or more, it increased to 1.601 (1.201–2.132), indicating a notable rise in IBTR rates over more extended observation periods. This suggests that breast-conserving therapy in young *BRCA1/2* mutation carriers carries a heightened risk of long-term IBTR.

However, these findings do not decisively argue against breast-conserving therapy for *BRCA1/2* mutation carriers, as IBTR may not solely result from radiation-induced cancer but could also stem from an underlying genetic predisposition to cancer. Although the risk is 1.6 times higher than in sporadic breast cancer, no significant difference in survival rates has been observed.

Therefore, the decision to undergo breast-conserving surgery with radiation therapy in *BRCA1/2* mutation carriers should be made following thorough patient counseling, considering the following factors: There is a potentially elevated risk of new breast cancer development in both the conserved and contralateral breasts.

IBTR rates increase with long-term follow-up.
Survival rates do not differ significantly compared to mastectomy.
Current clinical research data may have limitations.
IBTR may not always be detectable early.
Early-stage IBTR may necessitate chemotherapy.
Breast reconstruction post-radiotherapy is complex.

4.6.2 Risk-Reducing Mastectomies Are an Alternative Option: Breast Imaging Diagnosis Involving Radiation Exposure for BRCA1/2 *Mutation Carriers*

When considering appropriate imaging diagnostics, factors such as image quality controls—such as breast density by age, modality sensitivity, and radiation exposure—must be considered. Diagnostic radiation exposure varies, with reported doses of 0.06–0.11 mGy for plain X-rays, 10 mGy for whole-body CT scans, 7 mGy for chest CT scans, and 0.72 mGy for mammography [37]. Since ionizing radiation induces stochastic DNA damage, the risk of carcinogenesis increases with higher doses.

The GENE-RAD-RISK study, a large-scale retrospective cohort analysis [38], investigated the correlation between diagnostic radiological exams and breast cancer risk in *BRCA1/2* mutation carriers. It found a dose-dependent increase in breast cancer incidence, with a hazard ratio of 1.63 at a total radiation dose of 0.0020 Gy, equating to 0.0005 Gy for chest X-rays and 0.0042–0.0186 Gy for mammography. *BRCA1/2* mutation carriers exposed to radiation before age 30 had a 1.9-fold higher breast cancer risk compared to those without a radiation exposure history. However, no significant difference in breast cancer incidence was observed between groups exposed to radiation before age 40 versus before age 30, indicating that radiation exposure after age 30 did not significantly elevate risk.

It is important to note that self-reported radiation exposure history in the study may introduce recall bias, potentially inflating statements among new breast cancer patients. Few studies have examined the cumulative probabilistic effects of diagnostic radiation exposure on cancer development in *BRCA1/2* mutation carriers, and conclusive evidence remains lacking.

However, considering image accuracy, mammography exhibits a high false-negative rate for *BRCA1/2* mutation carriers and individuals with dense breasts [39]. Given that many individuals under age 30 have dense breasts, the utility of mammography screening is limited in this population. Consequently, current guidelines often do not recommend routine mammography for all *BRCA1/2* mutation carriers under age 30.

4.7 Conclusion

Recent interim results from an Israeli phase II clinical trial highlighted the incidence of contralateral breast cancer in early-stage *BRCA1/2* mutation carriers who underwent prophylactic radiation to the contralateral breast [40]. In this trial, 81 patients in the control arm received standard locoregional treatment, including surgery and radiation therapy to the affected side, while 81 patients in the intervention arm received additional contralateral breast irradiation. Over a median follow-up of 58 months, ten patients in the control arm developed contralateral breast cancer at a median of 32 months, whereas two patients in the intervention arm developed contralateral breast cancer at 80 and 105 months after bilateral breast irradiation (log-rank P = 0.011). Despite the global preference among *BRCA1/2* mutation carriers with unilateral breast cancer for bilateral mastectomy, these results from a clinical study provide valuable insights often overlooked. However, further studies are warranted due to the limited number of cases and the relatively short follow-up period.

The stochastic effect of radiation on developing secondary cancers in individuals carrying a germline *BRCA1/2* mutation in a single allele remains inconclusive. Continued accumulation and accurate interpretation of evidence are crucial for determining appropriate risk management strategies for each patient based on the cancer susceptibility of *BRCA1/2* mutation carriers. This decision-making process should consider medical evidence, precision, patient age, cosmetic outcomes, cost-effectiveness, and patient satisfaction.

References

1. World Health Organization 'Cancer Incidence in five continents volume XII'. Available at: https://ci5.iarc.fr/ci5-xii/. Accessed 26 May 2024.
2. Hristov B, Lin SH, Christodouleas JP. Radiation oncology: a question-based review. 3rd ed. Lippincott Williams & Wilkins; 2018.
3. Ministry of the Envoronment Government of Japan 'Booklet to provide basic information regarding health effects of radiation'. Available at: https://www.env.go.jp/chemi/rhm/r4kisoshiryo.html. Accessed 26 May 2024.
4. World Health Organization. Ionizing radiation, health effects and protective measures Apr 29 2016. Archived from the original on 29 March 2020. Retrieved 22 Jan 2020.
5. Bartek J, Bartkova J, Lukas J. DNA damage signalling guards against activated oncogenes and tumour progression. Oncogene 2007;26(56):7773–7779.
6. Vilenchik MM, Knudson AG. Endogenous DNA double-strand breaks: production, fidelity of repair, and induction of cancer. Proc Natl Acad Sci USA. 2003;100(22):12871–6.
7. Ciccia A, Elledge SJ. The DNA damage response: making it safe to play with knives. Mol Cell. 2010;40(2):179–204.
8. Maynard S, Schurman SH, Harboe C, de Souza-Pinto NC, Bohr VA. Base excision repair of oxidative DNA damage and association with cancer and aging. Carcinogenesis. 2009;30(1):2–10.
9. Shaltiel IA, Krenning L, Bruinsma W, Medema RH. The same, only different – DNA damage checkpoints and their reversal throughout the cell cycle. J Cell Sci. 2015;128(4):607–20.
10. Lakin ND, Jackson SP. Regulation of p53 in response to DNA damage. Oncogene. 1999;18(53):7644–55.
11. NCRP 2018 [online]. Commentary no. 27-implications of recent epidemiologic studies for the linear nonthreshold model and radiation protection Available at: https://www.ncrppublications.org/Commentaries/27. Accessed 3 May 2018.
12. Fanconi anemia Clinical Care Guidelines 5th 2020 Available at: https://fanconi.org/clinical-care-guidelines/clinical-care/. Accessed 26 May 2024.
13. Perlman S updated 2023 Nov 16. Hereditary ataxia overview. 1998 Oct 28. GeneReviews® [Internet]. In: Adam MP, Feldman J, Mirzaa GM, Pagon RA, Wallace SE, Bean LJH, Gripp KW, Amemiya A, editors. Seattle: University of Washington. Seattle; 1993–2024. Accessed 26 May 2024.

14. Bergom C, West CM, Higginson DS, et al. The implications of genetic testing on radiation therapy decisions: a guide for radiation oncologists. Int J Radiat Oncol Biol Phys. 2019;105(4):698–712.
15. Riaz N, Blecua P, Lim RS, et al. Pan-cancer analysis of bi-allelic alterations in homologous recombination DNA repair genes. Nat Commun. 2017;8(1):857.
16. Mutter RW, Riaz N, Ng CK, et al. Bi-allelic alterations in DNA repair genes underpin homologous recombination DNA repair defects in breast cancer. J Pathol. 2017;242(2):165–77.
17. NCCN clinical practice guidelines in oncology (NCCN Guidelines®) breast cancer version 3. 2024 Jun 17, 2024. Available at: https://www.nccn.org/.
18. Tung NM, Boughey JC, Pierce LJ, et al. Management of hereditary breast cancer: American Society of Clinical Oncology, American Society for Radiation Oncology, and Society of Surgical Oncology guideline. J Clin Oncol. 2020;38(18):2080–106.
19. Sessa C, Balmaña J, Bober SL, et al. Risk reduction and screening of cancer in hereditary breast-ovarian cancer syndromes: ESMO clinical practice guideline. Ann Oncol. 2023;34(1):33–47.
20. Manahan ER, Kuerer HM, Sebastian M, et al. Consensus guidelines on genetic` testing for hereditary breast cancer from the American Society of Breast Surgeons. Ann Surg Oncol. 2019;26(10):3025–31.
21. NCCN clinical practice guidelines in oncology (NCCN Guidelines®) genetic/familial high-risk assessment: breast, ovarian, and pancreatic version 3.2024 Feb 12, 2024 Available at: https://www.nccn.org/.
22. National Institute for Health and Care Excellence Available at: https://www.nice.org.uk/guidance. Accessed 26 May 2024.
23. Guidelines for diagnosis and treatment of hereditary breast and ovarian cancer 2021. Japanese Organization of Hereditary Breast and Ovarian Cancer Available at: https://johboc.jp/guidebook_2021/. Accessed 26 May 2024.
24. Garcia-Etienne CA, Barile M, Gentilini OD, et al. Breast—conserving surgery in BRCA1/2 mutation carriers:are we approaching an answer? Ann Surg Oncol. 2009;16(12):3380–7. [PMID:19649554].
25. Ye F, Huang L, Lang G, et al. Outcomes and risk of subsequent breast events in breast—conserving surgery patients with BRCA1 and BRCA2 mutation. Cancer Med. 2020;9(5):1903–10. [PMID:31912664].
26. Kirova YM, Savignoni A, Sigal-Zafrani B, et al. Is the breast—conserving treatment with radiotherapy appropriate in BRCA1/2 mutation carriers? Long—term results and review of the literature. Breast Cancer Res Treat. 2010;120(1):119–26. [PMID:20033769].
27. Yoon KH, Chae S, Kang E, et al. Contralateral breast cancer and ipsilateral breast tumor recurrence in BRCA1/2 carriers and non—carriers at high—risk of hereditary breast cancer. J Breast Cancer. 2019;22(4):587–98. [PMID:31897332].
28. Cao W, Xie Y, He Y, et al. Risk of ipsilateral breast tumor recurrence in primary invasive breast cancer following breast-conserving surgery with BRCA1 and BRCA2 mutation in China. Breast Cancer Res Treat. 2019;175(3):749–54. [PMID:30895535].
29. Pierce LJ, Strawderman M, Narod SA, et al. Effect of radiotherapy after breast—conserving treatment in women with breast cancer and germline BRCA1/2 mutations. J Clin Oncol. 2000;18(19):3360–9. [PMID:11013276].
30. El-Tamer M, Russo D, Troxel A, et al. Survival and recurrence after breast cancer in BRCA1/2 mutation carriers. Ann Surg Oncol. 2004;11(2):157–64. [PMID:14761918].
31. Robson ME, Chappuis PO, Satagopan J, et al. A combined analysis of outcome following breast cancer:differences in survival based on BRCA1/BRCA2 mutation status and administration of adjuvant treatment. Breast Cancer Res. 2004;6(1):R8–R17. [PMID:14680495].
32. Pierce LJ, Levin AM, Rebbeck TR, et al. Ten—year multi—institutional results of breast—conserving surgery and radiotherapy in BRCA1/2—associated stage I/II breast cancer. J Clin Oncol. 2006;24(16):2437–43. [PMID:16636335].

33. Seynaeve C, Verhoog LC, van de Bosch LM, et al. Ipsilateral breast tumour recurrence in hereditary breast cancer following breast—conserving therapy. Eur J Cancer. 2004;40(8):1150–8. [PMID:15110878].
34. Eccles D, Simmonds P, Goddard J, et al. Familial breast cancer: an investigation into the outcome of treatment for early stage disease. Fam Cancer. 2001;1(2):65–72. [PMID:14573999].
35. Haffty BG, Harrold E, Khan AJ, et al. Outcome of conservatively managed early—onset breast cancer by BRCA1/2 status. Lancet. 2002;359(9316):1471–7. [PMID:11988246].
36. Robson M, Gilewski T, Haas B, et al. BRCA—associated breast cancer in young women. J Clin Oncol. 1998;16(5):1642–9. [PMID:9586873].
37. Mettler FA Jr, Bhargavan M, Faulkner K, et al. Radiologic and nuclear medicine studies in the United States and worldwide: frequency, radiation dose, and comparison with other radiation sources-1950-2007. Radiology. 2009;253(2):520–31.
38. Pijpe A, Andrieu N, Easton DF, et al. GENEPSO; embrace; HEBON. Exposure to diagnostic radiation and risk of breast cancer among carriers of BRCA1/2 mutations: retrospective cohort study(GENE-RAD-RISK). BMJ. 2012;345:e5660.
39. Tilanus-Linthorst M, Verhoog L, Obdeijn IM, et al. A BRCA1/2 mutation, high breast density and prominent pushing margins of a tumor independently contribute to a frequent false-negative mammography. Int J Cancer. 2002;102(1):91–5.
40. Evron E, Ben-David AM, Goldberg H, et al. Prophylactic irradiation to the contralateral breast for BRCA mutation carriers with early-stage breast cancer. Ann Oncol. 2019;30(3):412–7.

Chapter 5
Why Is There a Difference in Age at Breast Cancer Onset Between *BRCA1* and *BRCA2* Carriers?

Tomoyuki Aruga

5.1 Background

The presence of germline pathogenic variants of *BRCA1* or *BRCA2* is called hereditary breast and ovarian cancer (HBOC), and the lifetime incidence of breast, ovarian, and related cancers is known to be higher in patients with these variants than in the general population. Both the *BRCA1* and *BRCA2* are genes related to homologous recombination repair, and homologous recombination deficiency (HRD) is known to occur in the absence of these genes. However, there are differences in subtypes and the age at onset of breast cancer between *BRCA1* and *BRCA2* variant carriers. This chapter discusses the difference in age at the onset of breast cancer among carriers of BRCA1 and 2 pathogenic variants and the cause of this discrepancy.

5.1.1 Differences in Cumulative Breast Cancer Incidence Between BRCA1 and BRCA2

A meta-analysis of ten reports published in 2007 found that the cumulative incidence of breast cancer in *BRCA1* and *BRCA2* pathogenic variant carriers in their 30s, 40s, 50s, 60s, and 70s was 1.8% and 1%, 12% and 7.5%, 29% and 21%, 44% and 35%, and 54% and 45%, respectively. The difference in the breast cancer incidence rate between these groups emerged by 50 years of age [1]. To exclude the effect of risk-reducing salpingo-oophorectomy (RRSO) on the breast cancer

T. Aruga (✉)
Department of Breast Surgery, Surgical Specialities, Institute of Science Tokyo, Tokyo, Japan

T. Ohta et al. (eds.), *Practical Guide to Hereditary Breast and Ovarian Cancer III*, https://doi.org/10.1007/978-981-96-6779-6_5

incidence, a meta-analysis of breast cancer incidence in an HBOC population not receiving RRSO found that the cumulative incidence of breast cancer among *BRCA1* and *BRCA2* pathogenic variant carriers in their 30s, 40s, 50s, 60s, 707s, and 80s was 2.9% and 2.5%,19.2% and 13.5%, 39.5% and 31.5%, 52.5% and 47.5%, 64.6% and 61.0%, and 69.2% and 66.9%, respectively [2]. Furthermore, a prospective cohort study of 6036 *BRCA1* and 3820 *BRCA2* pathogenic variant carriers recruited between 1997 and 2011 reported a cumulative breast cancer incidence rate in their 20s, 30s, 40s, 50s, 60s, and 70s as 4% and 4%, 24% and 13%, 43% and 35%, 56% and 53%, 66% and 61%, and 72% and 69, respectively. These findings also indicate that the difference in the breast cancer incidence between *BRCA1* and *BRCA2* pathogenic variant carriers generally emerged by the age of 50 years [3]. These data suggest that the difference in the breast cancer incidence associated with *BRCA1* and *BRCA2* is largely due to more breast cancers occurring in individuals with a *BRCA1* pathogenic variant than in those with a *BRCA2* pathogenic variant before the age of 50 years (Fig. 5.1).

5.1.2 BRCA1 Pathogenic Variants and Subtypes of Breast Cancer

Of the breast cancer subtypes developing in carriers of *BRCA1* pathogenic variants, triple negative breast cancer (TNBC) had an incidence of 65%, which was much higher than in the general population [4] (Fig. 5.2). A study of 35,000 patients with breast cancer found that germline pathogenic variants of 25 inherited tumor-related genes, including 12 breast cancer predisposition genes, were detected in 9.3% of the patients; of these, *BRCA1* and *BRCA2* accounted for 24% and 24.4%, respectively. Considering that the positivity rate was higher in patients with TNBC younger than 50 years (18.4%) than in patients with no TNBC (9.5%) and that *BRCA1 and 2* are the most common causative genes in positive individuals younger than 40 years, the difference in breast cancer incidence between carriers of pathogenic *BRCA1* and *BRCA2* variants is presumably due mainly to TNBC occurring in *BRCA1* by the age of 50 years [5] (Fig. 5.3).

5.1.3 Association of TNBC and Female Hormones in BRCA1 Carriers

The incidence of TNBC after RRSO in premenopausal *BRCA1* pathogenic variant carriers is useful for determining the extent to which female hormones are involved in TNBC development. A meta-analysis of breast cancer incidence after RRSO in HBOC reported a reduction in the breast cancer incidence among patients with RRSO regardless of whether the patients had had breast cancer previously. In the

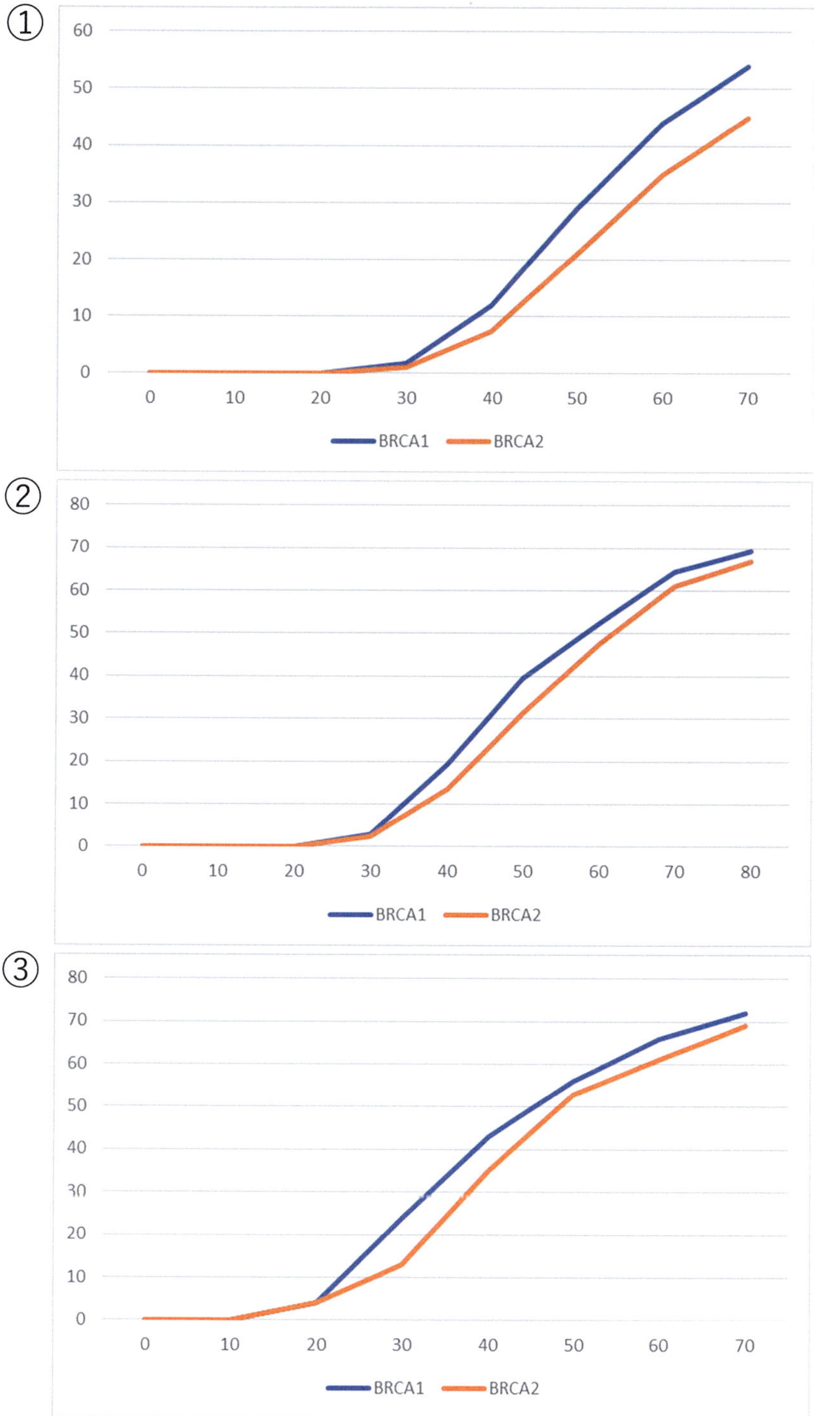

Fig. 5.1 Breast cancer cumulative incidence rate. Drawing based on data from the above three reports [1–3]

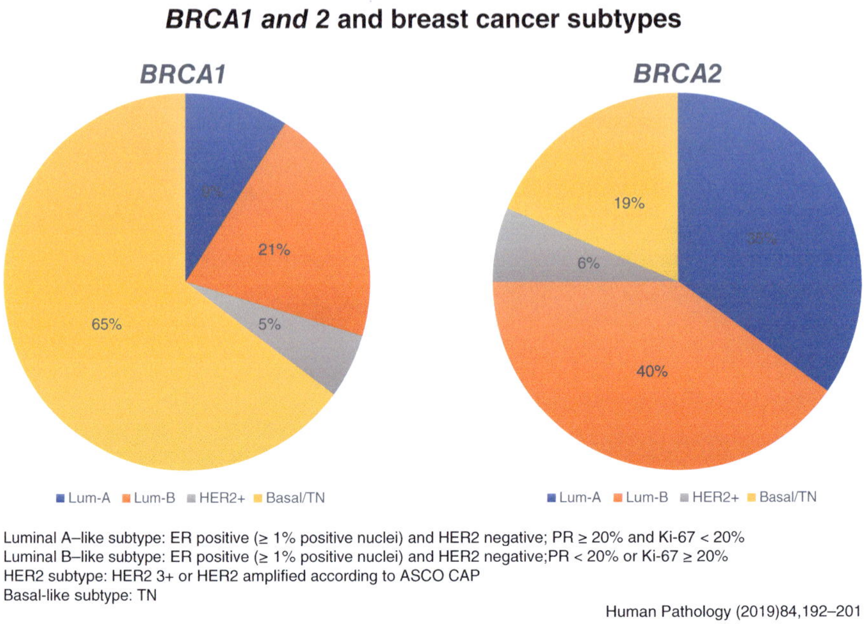

Fig. 5.2 *BRCA1/2* and breast cancer subtypes

breast cancer-free group, there was no significant difference in breast cancer risk reduction by RRSO between *BRCA1* and *BRCA2* (*BRCA1,* HR: 0.65; 95% confidence interval [CI]: 0.42–0.87; *BRCA2,* HR: 0.53; 95% CI: 0.33–0.74). These findings suggested that RRSO may suppress breast cancer development in carriers of either a *BRCA1* or *BRCA2* pathogenic variant. Furthermore, the greater reduction in breast cancer risk with RRSO at age < 50 years (< 50 years, HR: 0.45; 95% CI: 0.24–0.67; > 50 years, HR: 0.83; 95% CI: 0.01–1.66) suggested that the effect of RRSO on reducing this risk was associated with lower female hormone levels [6].

The involvement of female hormones in TNBC developing in HBOC can be inferred from the frequency of breast cancer in relation to hormone replacement therapy (HRT) following RRSO. A cohort study enrolling 462 women with a germline pathogenic variant of *BRCA1* or *BRCA2* evaluated the breast cancer risk associated with HRT after RRSO and found no significant change in relation to any form of HRT [7]. However, a 2018 study focusing on *BRCA1* pathogenic variant carriers reported an increased risk of breast cancer (HR: 1.64; 95% CI: 0.68–3.98) when hormone replacement was performed with estrogen (E) plus progesterone (P) after RRSO at age < 45 years but not when E was administered alone (HR: 0.47; 95% CI: 0.20–1.15), suggesting that P-containing HRT increased the breast cancer risk in *BRCA1* pathogenic variant carriers who underwent RRSO [8].

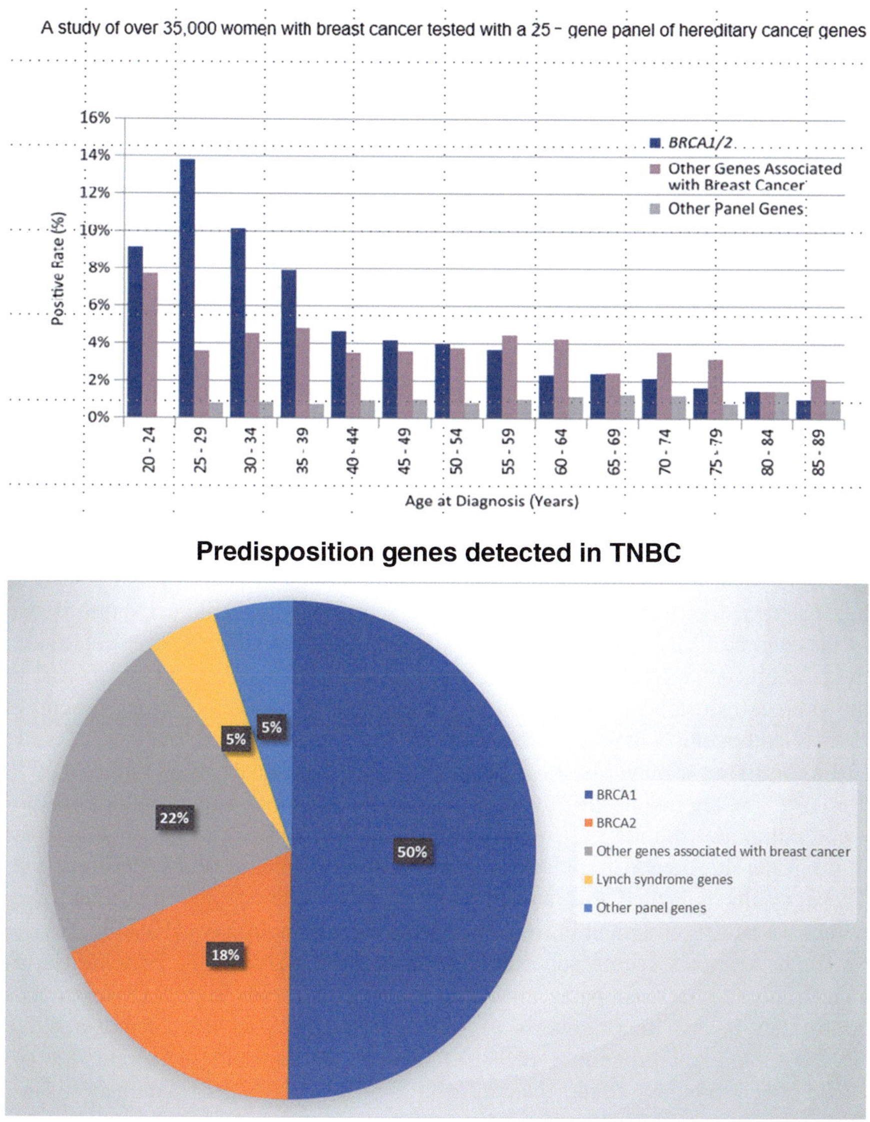

Cancer. 2017 May 15;123(10):1721-1730

Fig. 5.3 Predisposition gene rate by age and predisposition genes detected in TNBC

5.1.4 Mechanism of TNBC Development in BRCA1 Pathogenic Variant Carriers

The development of TNBC is thought to involve the oncogenic transformation of ER-/PR- luminal progenitor cells that have differentiated from common luminal progenitor cells [9]. This raises the question of whether progesterone is involved in the transformation of *BRCA1*$^{mut/+}$ ER-/PR- luminal progenitors into basal-like cancer cells.

In experiments using *Brca1*$^{f/f}$*p53*$^{f/f}$ conditional knockout mice, in which the pathogenic variants of *BRCA1* and *p53* occur in the mammary tissue, proliferative changes in mammary gland morphology, such as ductal branching, lobule formation, and high proliferative potential often observed during pregnancy, reportedly occurred at a higher rate in *Brca1*$^{f/f}$*p53*$^{f/f}$ mammary tissue than in wild-type mammary tissue or mammary tissue with only the *p53* pathogenic variant (p53$^{f/f}$). In addition, the simultaneous administration of estradiol (E2) and progesterone (P4) to *Brca1*$^{f/f}$*p53*$^{f/f}$ mice overactivated cell proliferation in mammary tissue compared to either E2 or P4 alone. Furthermore, *Brca1*$^{f/f}$*p53*$^{f/f}$ mice reportedly demonstrated progesterone receptor expression in almost all the mammary tissue during the estrous phase, suggesting that progesterone-induced mammary epithelial activation is one of the causes of carcinogenesis in *BRCA1*-inactivated mammary tissue. This raises the possibility that ER-/PR- luminal progenitor cells are transformed into TNBC in the premenopausal, estradiol- and progesterone-rich, hormonal environment in *BRCA1* pathogenic variant carriers.

Furthermore, a previous study found that all nonpregnant mice with *Brca1*$^{f11/f11}$*p53*$^{f5\&6/f5\&6}$Crec in a no-treatment or placebo group demonstrated tumor development within nine months, whereas a group treated with mifepristone, an antagonist of progesterone, demonstrated complete suppression of breast cancer development. These results indicated that antagonizing progesterone before menopause may reduce TNBC development in *BRCA1* pathogenic variant carriers [10] (Fig. 5.4).

Tumor necrosis factor superfamily member 11 (TNFSF11, also known as RANKL), an important paracrine effector of progesterone signaling, reportedly contributes to the tumorigenesis of *BRCA1*$^{mut/+}$ cells, and its receptor-positive (RANK+) luminal progenitor cells (LPs) were significantly more abundant in *BRCA1*$^{mut/+}$ mammary tissue than in wild type or *BRCA2*$^{mut/+}$ mammary tissue. RANK+ LP are mitotically active and prone to DNA damage, suggesting a process by which RANK+ ER-/PR- LPs can become cancerous in *BRCA1*$^{mut/+}$ mammary tissue. Furthermore, treatment with denosumab, an anti-RANKL monoclonal antibody, strongly suppresses tumor onset in *BRCA1*-deficient mice, suggesting that denosumab may suppress breast cancer development in *BRCA1* pathogenic variant carriers [11]. Clinical validation of the BRCA-P study is currently underway (Fig. 5.5).

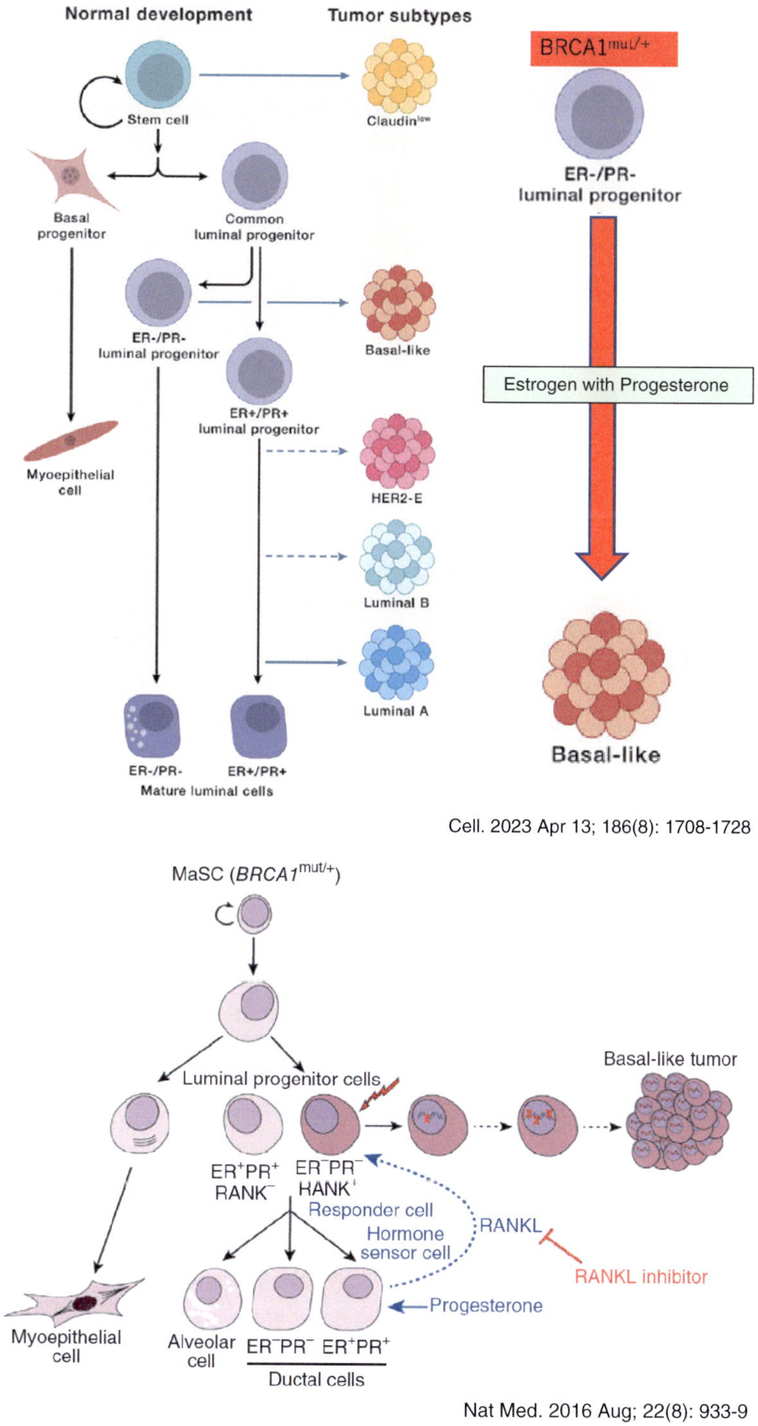

Fig. 5.4 Pathogenesis of basal-like tumors and involvement of progesterone and RANKL

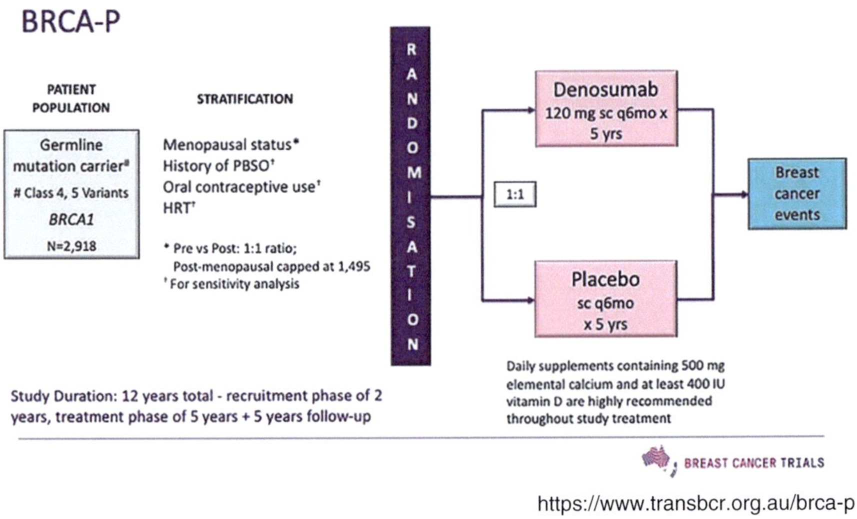

Fig. 5.5 BRCA-P study design

5.2 Conclusion

The difference in the cumulative breast cancer incidence observed between *BRCA1* and *2* pathogenic variant carriers may be due to a higher incidence of premenopausal TNBC in *BRCA1* carriers, and molecules such as progesterone and RANKL may be closely involved in this oncogenic process. Drugs targeting these molecules have the potential to prevent TNBC development in *BRCA1* carriers.

References

1. Chen S, Parmigiani G. Meta-analysis of BRCA1 and BRCA2 penetrance. J Clin Oncol. 2007;25(11):1329–33.
2. Chen J, Bae E, Zhang L, Hughes K, Parmigiani G, Braun D, et al. Penetrance of breast and ovarian cancer in women who carry a BRCA1/2 mutation and do not use risk-reducing Salpingo-oophorectomy: an updated meta-analysis. JNCI Cancer Spectr. 2020;4(4):pkaa029.
3. Kuchenbaecker KB, Hopper JL, Barnes DR, Phillips KA, Mooij TM, Roos-Blom MJ, et al. Risks of breast, ovarian, and contralateral breast cancer for BRCA1 and BRCA2 mutation carriers. JAMA. 2017;317(23):2402–16.
4. Sonderstrup IMH, Jensen MR, Ejlertsen B, Eriksen JO, Gerdes AM, Kruse TA, et al. Subtypes in BRCA-mutated breast cancer. Hum Pathol. 2019;84:192–201.
5. Buys SS, Sandbach JF, Gammon A, Patel G, Kidd J, Brown KL, et al. A study of over 35,000 women with breast cancer tested with a 25-gene panel of hereditary cancer genes. Cancer. 2017;123(10):1721–30.

6. Xiao YL, Wang K, Liu Q, Li J, Zhang X, Li HY. Risk reduction and survival benefit of risk-reducing Salpingo-oophorectomy in hereditary breast cancer: meta-analysis and systematic review. Clin Breast Cancer. 2019;19(1):e48–65.
7. Rebbeck TR, Friebel T, Wagner T, Lynch HT, Garber JE, Daly MB, et al. Effect of short-term hormone replacement therapy on breast cancer risk reduction after bilateral prophylactic oophorectomy in BRCA1 and BRCA2 mutation carriers: the PROSE study group. J Clin Oncol. 2005;23(31):7804–10.
8. Kotsopoulos J, Gronwald J, Karlan BY, Huzarski T, Tung N, Moller P, et al. Hormone replacement therapy after oophorectomy and breast cancer risk among BRCA1 mutation carriers. JAMA Oncol. 2018;4(8):1059–65.
9. Nolan E, Lindeman GJ, Visvader JE. Deciphering breast cancer: from biology to the clinic. Cell. 2023;186(8):1708–28.
10. Poole AJ, Li Y, Kim Y, Lin SC, Lee WH, Lee EY. Prevention of Brca1-mediated mammary tumorigenesis in mice by a progesterone antagonist. Science. 2006;314(5804):1467–70.
11. Nolan E, Vaillant F, Branstetter D, Pal B, Giner G, Whitehead L, et al. RANK ligand as a potential target for breast cancer prevention in BRCA1-mutation carriers. Nat Med. 2016;22(8):933–9.

Part III
Preimplantation Genetic Testing

Chapter 6
Clinical Ethical Issues Regarding Hereditary Breast Cancer and Ovarian Cancer Syndrome and the Preimplantation Genetic Test for a Monogenic/Single-Gene Defect in Japan

Nao Suzuki

6.1 Oncofertility

Oncofertility is an interdisciplinary medical field that bridges biomedicine and social sciences and examines issues related to individual patients' fertility options, decisions, and goals with respect to a cancer diagnosis, treatment, and survivorship. Clinically, oncofertility aims to achieve physical, mental, and social well-being for cancer patients of reproductive or pre-reproductive age by providing assistance based on biomedicine and social sciences to enable patients and their families to have children and/or to reexamine what it means to have children. In Japan, the Japan Society for Fertility Preservation was established in 2012, and in 2014, the Japan Society of Obstetrics and Gynecology (JSOG) officially stated its views on medically indicated cryopreservation. Three years later, in 2017, the Japan Society of Clinical Oncology (JSCO) published the "JSCO Clinical Practice Guidelines 2017 for Fertility Preservation in Childhood, Adolescent and Young Adult Cancer Patients" [1, 2].

Fertility preservation and cancer treatment put such a large financial burden on patients with cancer aged 0–39 years and their families that many of them, including adolescent and young adult (AYA) patients (age range, 15–39 years), are forced to give up undergoing fertility preservation therapy. Against this backdrop, in April 2021, the government initiated a financial support program related to fertility preservation that amounted to 22 billion yen (Cancer and Disease Control Division, Ministry of Health, Labour and Welfare: The Research Promotion of Fertility Preservation for Childhood and AYA Generation Cancer Patients). This program

N. Suzuki (✉)
Department of Obstetrics and Gynecology, St. Marianna University School of Medicine, Kawasaki, Kanagawa, Japan
e-mail: nao@marianna-u.ac.jp

T. Ohta et al. (eds.), *Practical Guide to Hereditary Breast and Ovarian Cancer III*, https://doi.org/10.1007/978-981-96-6779-6_6

offered great hope to patients with cancer and their families, especially those who could not afford fertility preservation therapy. Later, in March 2023, the Cabinet approved the "Basic Plan to Promote Cancer Control Programs (4th-term basic plan)," which included the new item "Fertility preservation therapy" under "(1) Systems for provision of cancer care" as one of the "Cancer Care" section goals aimed at improving the quality of life in survivorship of both cancer patients and their families. These national cancer control programs related to fertility preservation are highly beneficial to childhood and AYA patients with cancer who must continue living with the disease.

As described above, oncofertility is making significant advances in Japan. When providing decision-making support to patients and their families before the start of cancer treatment, it is important that healthcare professionals listen to patients' and families' wishes regarding fertility preservation, including the available options if they decide against fertility preservation. To this end, establishing a decision-making support system that facilitates the provision of reliable information at the right time is crucial. Above all, there is an urgent need for further education and training among healthcare professionals involved in oncofertility to ensure that while prioritizing cancer treatment, they also provide decision-making support to patients with cancer and their families, who are anxious and fearful as they deal with uncertainty in the future (Fig. 6.1).

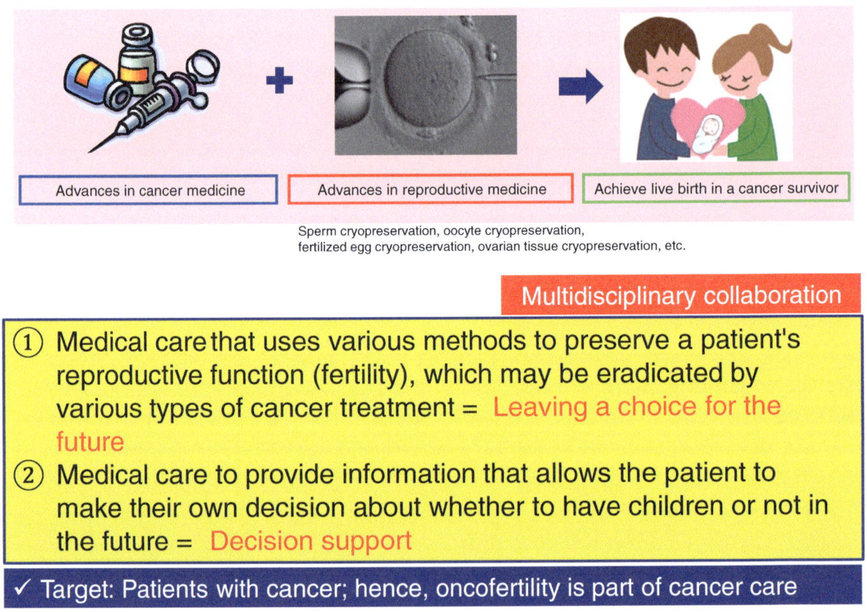

Fig. 6.1 What is oncofertility?

6.2 Views of the JSOG and the Preimplantation Genetic Test for a Monogenic/Single-Gene Defect

In the roughly 40 years since publication in 1983 of the JSOG's views on in vitro fertilization and embryo transfer, the JSOG has asked its members to conform to its views and opinions on ethically sensitive matters. The following text regarding matters requiring ethical consideration in clinical and research practices is posted on the website of the JSOG: "The JSOG advocates for clinical and research activities that are conducted with full ethical consideration in light of recent social situations. To this end, the JSOG has published guidelines to present its views on ethically sensitive matters in clinical and research practices. Here, these views are presented together once again for the convenience of members and for the purpose of urging members to take particular care regarding these matters. We request that our members strictly conform to these views when conducting clinical and research activities. Members who fail to conform to the society's views will be subject to prompt and careful investigation of the circumstances, with appropriate action taken in accordance with the standing rules if necessary." It should be noted that the views and opinions of the JSOG, which are more or less agreements between the general public and obstetrics and gynecology physicians who provide care, including reproductive medicine services, are purely self-regulatory in nature and that the JSOG does not have the power to control the actions of physicians who are not JSOG members. In other words, the regulations are not legally binding, which is problematic.

A preimplantation genetic test for a monogenic/single-gene defect (PGT-M) was performed for the first time in 1992 in the United Kingdom for the preimplantation diagnosis of cystic fibrosis disease gene carriers. In response to the introduction of this testing, the JSOG published its "Views on Preimplantation Genetic Testing for Serious Genetic Diseases" in 1998, and PGT-M was approved for the first time in 2004 for use in a patient with Duchenne muscular dystrophy. The JSOG defined a "serious genetic disease," when used to describe the circumstances under which PGT-M may be applicable, as "a condition in which symptoms appear that significantly impair daily living or threaten the survival of the patient before they reach adulthood." This definition remained standing for a long time; however, in 2018, a JSOG committee did not approve a reapplication for PGT-M by a patient with retinoblastoma, which led to further discussions as to what the definition of a "serious genetic disease" should entail in the context of PGT-M. Although symptoms of retinoblastoma appear before patients reach adulthood, PGT-M was not approved for use in the patient with retinoblastoma because the disease is not life-threatening and is not associated with symptoms that significantly impair a patient's daily life. However, blindness due to retinoblastoma is considered serious because it significantly impairs daily life, and although the treatment outcome of the primary disease is generally favorable, patient survival and prognosis are affected by whether there is an onset of secondary cancer and by the success or failure of the treatment of such a cancer. Accordingly, strong arguments were made for the need for social consensus and for fully considering a person's feelings. This debate underscored yet again the importance of clinical ethical discussions, which should take into full account both individuals' rights to pursue happiness and the rejection of eugenics. The JSOG determined that the standards and processes used to review the applicability of PGT-M and judge whether to approve or disapprove its use, which relied only on medical criteria, would need to be reconsidered. Thus, with the aim to widely review opinions and reach social consensus, the JSOG held a total of three ethics council meetings on PGT-M from 2020 to 2021. These meetings were attended by a diverse range of professionals, who selected committee members, and by many observer groups and members of the public because the meetings also served as public lectures. As a consequence of these meetings, the JSOG redefined a "serious genetic disease" with respect to PGT-M as the following: "as a general principle, a condition in which symptoms that significantly impair the daily life of the patient appear before reaching adulthood or in which the survival of the patient is threatened and for which either there is no effective treatment to avoid these risks at the present moment or advanced and highly invasive treatment is required" (January 2022). The JSOG also reviewed the method for screening patients.

In the meantime, the sectional committee to discuss issues related to preimplantation diagnosis, specifically PGT-M, of the Science Council of Japan Section II (Chairperson, Tomoyuki Fujii; Vice-Chairperson, Noriko Mizuno) took the lead and conducted seven deliberations. Subsequently, in August 2023, the committee issued the recommendations, termed "Establishment of a public platform for the proper operation of preimplantation genetic testing (PGT) with ethical challenges—with a focus on the handling of PGT-M for genetic disorders." The recommendations include a statement that a public institution needs to be established that is responsible for examining reproductive medicine, including PGT-M and bioethics, and for deliberating on, agreeing on, and standardizing bioethics "related to medical care enabling babies to be born." Today, with advances in genomic medicine and in response to the steady and rapid progress of medical technologies, it is imperative that a system is constructed that allows for the provision of high-quality medical care to patients by continuing discussions and obtaining social consensus. Although the term "serious genetic disease," which determines the applicability of PGT-M, was redefined for the first time in 18 years, there remains a need to continue the deliberations, e.g., on the definition of "serious genetic disease" from the perspective of clinical ethics.

6.3 "Research Promotion of Fertility Preservation for Childhood and AYA Generation Cancer Patients" and Future Issues (PGT-M)

The "Research Promotion of Fertility Preservation for Childhood and AYA Generation Cancer Patients," which was launched in Japan in 2021, must solve three issues that are expected to arise in the future: 1. cancer during pregnancy, 2. posthumous assisted reproduction, and 3. measures related to PGT-M for hereditary breast cancer and ovarian cancer syndrome (HBOC) (Fig. 6.2).

HBOC is a syndrome that makes it more likely that a person will develop germline *BRCA* pathogenic variant-associated cancer, including breast, ovarian, prostate, and pancreatic cancers. Hereditary neoplasms related to such a cancer predisposition are due to mutations in single genes and have been reported to account for 7–10% of breast cancer cases [3]. Currently, with advances in fertility preservation therapy, many cryopreserved embryos exist that carry *BRCA1/2* pathogenic variants, but technically, it is possible avoid passing on the disease by using PGT-M to select unaffected embryos. However, in Japan, the use of PGT-M to identify embryos with HBOC risk has never been approved because of the interpretation of a "serious genetic disease." As mentioned above, PGT-M, which enables the avoidance and elimination of diseases, must be examined from a multifaceted perspective that considers ethical, legal, and social issues. HBOC has a low penetration rate and does not result in a situation where the daily life of the patient is severely impaired by the

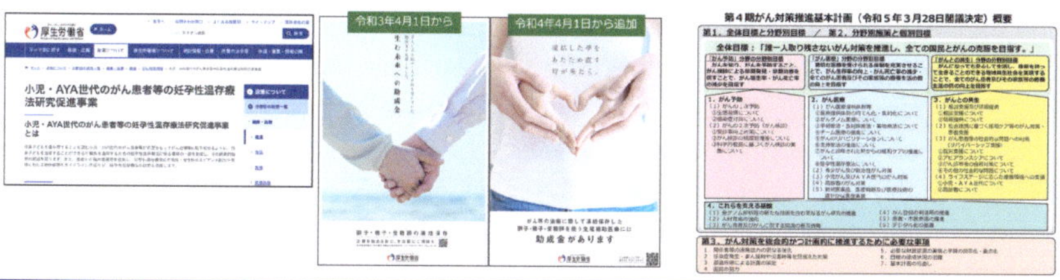

✓ Issues that are expected to arise in the future and therefore require solutions (by putting measures in place)

1. **Cancer during pregnancy (e.g., breast cancer)**
2. **Posthumous assisted reproduction**
3. **Preimplantation genetic test for a monogenic/single - gene defect (PGT-M) for hereditary breast and ovarian cancer syndrome**

Fig. 6.2 Research promotion of fertility preservation for childhood and AYA generation cancer patients (from 2021)

onset of symptoms or the patient's survival is threatened before they reach adulthood. Moreover, at present, effective treatments are available to avoid such a situation (e.g., genetic testing and preventive surgery, including risk-reducing salpingo-oophorectomy and risk-reducing mastectomy); therefore, it appears to be correct that HBOC is not included in the medical indications for PGT-M defined on the basis of the new definition of a "serious genetic disease." On the other hand, in some countries outside Japan, PGT-M is considered ethically acceptable for adult-onset monogenic disorders in terms of "freedom in reproduction" [4, 5]. Furthermore, some academic groups in the United States argue that genetic testing of fetuses and fertilized eggs (or embryos) for adult-onset diseases without a subsequent preventive intervention is a violation of a child's right to be free from knowledge about its genetic information and is inappropriate. On the other hand, the results of an evaluation of the cost-effectiveness of PGT-M from the aspect of social issues showed that PGT-M to identify *BRCA* pathogenic variant carriers is in fact cost-effective [6, 7]. In Japan, since the launch of the Research Promotion of Fertility Preservation for Childhood and AYA Generation Cancer Patients, an increasing number of patients with early-onset breast cancer have undergone cryopreservation of unfertilized or fertilized eggs as a means of fertility preservation. Given the proportion of HBOC cases in early-onset breast cancer, it is expected that in the future, some patients with early-onset breast cancer may wish to undergo PGT-M of their cryopreserved samples. Therefore, in Japan, there is an urgent need for discussions on the definition of the term "serious genetic disease" as it relates to the indications for PGT-M. However, so far, Japan has not provided a place for discussion and debate aimed at obtaining social consensus where experts in various fields and concerned parties come together to discuss the ethical, legal, and social implications of reproductive medicine. As mentioned above, the JSOG has been working to "provide high-quality and appropriate assisted reproductive medicine," which is the responsibility of physicians, by making public the views of the JSOG. Meanwhile, Article 4 ("Responsibility of the State") of the "Act on Assisted Reproductive Technology Offering and the Special Provisions of the Civil Code Related to the Parent-Child Relationship of a Child Born As a Result of the Treatment" issued in December 2020 includes statements such as "(1) Taking into consideration the basic principles set forth in the preceding Article, the State has the responsibility to formulate and implement a comprehensive policy to ensure appropriate offering of assisted reproductive technology" and "(2) In conducting the policy formulation and implementation referred to in the preceding paragraph, the State must take bioethics into consideration and must try to obtain the understanding of the people." "The understanding of the people" equates to social consensus, and to realize the state's responsibility to take "bioethics into consideration" and try "to obtain the understanding of the people," it is imperative that a public control organization is established; however, discussions about establishing such an organization have long been neglected. Furthermore, Article 6 "Dissemination of Knowledge" and Article 7 "Establishment of Consultation System" are included in the Act on Special Provisions to the Civil Code, and the need for legislative measures is clearly stated in Article 8, as follows: "...the State must take necessary legislative and other measures in order to ensure appropriate offerings, etc., of assisted reproductive technology." However, as of September 2023, i.e., about three years since the issuance of the Act on Special Provisions to the Civil Code, legislative and other measures necessary to ensure the appropriate provision of assisted reproductive medicine to the Japanese population are yet to be taken. This situation must be resolved as soon as possible. For roughly 40 years, the JSOG has called on its members to conform to the society's views and opinions on ethically sensitive matters. Efforts have also been directed toward facilitating the provision of high-quality and appropriate assisted reproductive health care. The government should clarify its responsibilities and those of healthcare professionals as soon as possible. The JSOG strongly requests that, in collaboration with the national government, a public platform is established to discuss, supervise, and manage bioethics related to medical care in the reproductive and perinatal periods. The society also highlights the pressing need in Japan for discussions on the definition of the term "serious genetic disease" as it relates to the indications for PGT-M.

References

1. Harada M, Kimura F, Takai Y, Nakajima T, Ushijima K, Kobayashi H, Satoh T, Tozawa A, Sugimoto K, Saji S, Shimizu C, Akiyama K, Bando H, Kuwahara A, Furui T, Okada H, Kawai K, Shinohara N, Nagao K, Kitajima M, Suenobu S, Soejima T, Miyachi M, Miyoshi Y, Yoneda A, Horie A, Ishida Y, Usui N, Kanda Y, Fujii N, Endo M, Nakayama R, Hoshi M, Yonemoto T, Kiyotani C, Okita N, Baba E, Muto M, Kikuchi I, Morishige KI, Tsugawa K, Nishiyama H, Hosoi H, Tanimoto M, Kawai A, Sugiyama K, Boku N, Yonemura M, Hayashi N, Aoki D, Osuga Y, Suzuki N. Japan Society of Clinical Oncology Clinical Practice Guidelines 2017 for fertility preservation in childhood, adolescent, and young adult cancer patients: part 1. Int J Clin Oncol. 2022;27:265–80.
2. Tozawa A, Kimura F, Takai Y, Nakajima T, Ushijima K, Kobayashi H, Satoh T, Harada M, Sugimoto K, Saji S, Shimizu C, Akiyama K, Bando H, Kuwahara A, Furui T, Okada H, Kawai K, Shinohara N, Nagao K, Kitajima M, Suenobu S, Soejima T, Miyachi M, Miyoshi Y, Yoneda A, Horie A, Ishida Y, Usui N, Kanda Y, Fujii N, Endo M, Nakayama R, Hoshi M, Yonemoto T, Kiyotani C, Okita N, Baba E, Muto M, Kikuchi I, Morishige KI, Tsugawa K, Nishiyama H, Hosoi H, Tanimoto M, Kawai A, Sugiyama K, Boku N, Yonemura M, Hayashi N, Aoki D, Suzuki N, Osuga Y. Japan Society of Clinical Oncology Clinical Practice Guidelines 2017 for fertility preservation in childhood, adolescent, and young adult cancer patients: part 2. Int J Clin Oncol. 2022;27:281–300.
3. Kauff ND. Management of BRCA-Negative Herediatry Breast Cancer Families. Hereditary Breast Cancer (Claudine Isaacs C, Rebbeck TR), CRC Press. 2007; pp 311–18.
4. Shenfield F, Pennings G, Devroey P, Sureau C, Tarlatzis B, Cohen J; ESHRE Ethics Task Force. Taskforce 5: preimplantation genetic diagnosis. Hum Reprod. 2003;3:649–51.
5. Ethics Committee of the American Society for Reproductive Medicine. Electronic address. Use of preimplantation genetic testing for monogenic defects (PGT-M) for adult-onset conditions: an Ethics Committee opinion. Fertil Steril. 2018;109:989–92.
6. Lipton JH, Zargar M, Warner E, Greenblatt EE, Lee E, Chan KKW, William Wong WWL. Cost effectiveness of in vitro fertilisation and preimplantation genetic testing to prevent transmission of BRCA1/2 mutations. Hum Reprod. 2020;35:434–45.
7. Michaan N, Leshno M, Cohen Y, Safra T, Peleg-Hasson S, Laskov I, Grisaru D. Preimplantation genetic testing for BRCA gene mutation carriers: a cost effectiveness analysis. Reprod Biol Endcrinol. 2021;19:153.

Chapter 7
Comments on the HBOC Guideline for PGT-M in Japan

Aiko Sasaki

Abstract In Japan, detailed discussions on the indication for preimplantation genetic testing for monogenic disorders (PGT-M), i.e., "which couples are justified to undergo PGT-M," have just begun. At present, PGT-M for low penetration or late-onset hereditary disease, such as hereditary breast and ovarian cancer (HBOC), is not publicly allowed domestically. Globally, although PGT-M for HBOC is already being implemented, it is not systematically recommended in the guidelines. Thus, its handling remains a controversial area not only from a medical standpoint but also from a bioethical perspective.

Keywords Preimplantation genetic testing for monogenic disorders (PGT-M) · Japan Society of Obstetricians and Gynecology (JSOG) · Maternal Health Act · Eugenics

7.1 Introduction

Regarding the statement on Japanese HBOC Clinical Guidelines BQ10 for the 2021 edition [6], "How should genetic counseling regarding reproduction be dealt with?," it was decided that "Although the option of preimplantation genetic testing for monogenic disorders (PGT-M) may arise for individuals with *BRCA1/2* pathogenic variants, at present, HBOC is not approved to be the indication of PGT-M based on the interpretation of its severity within the Japan Society of Obstetrics and Gynecology." We will explain the background of this decision.

At present, the term "preimplantation diagnosis" has been changed to "preimplantation genetic testing" by the Japan Society of Obstetrics and Gynecology as a specialized terminology.

A. Sasaki (✉)
Center for Maternal-Fetal, Neonatal and Reproductive Medicine/Center for Medical Genetics, National Center for Child Health and Development, Tokyo, Japan
e-mail: sasaki-a@ncchd.go.jp

T. Ohta et al. (eds.), *Practical Guide to Hereditary Breast and Ovarian Cancer III*, https://doi.org/10.1007/978-981-96-6779-6_7

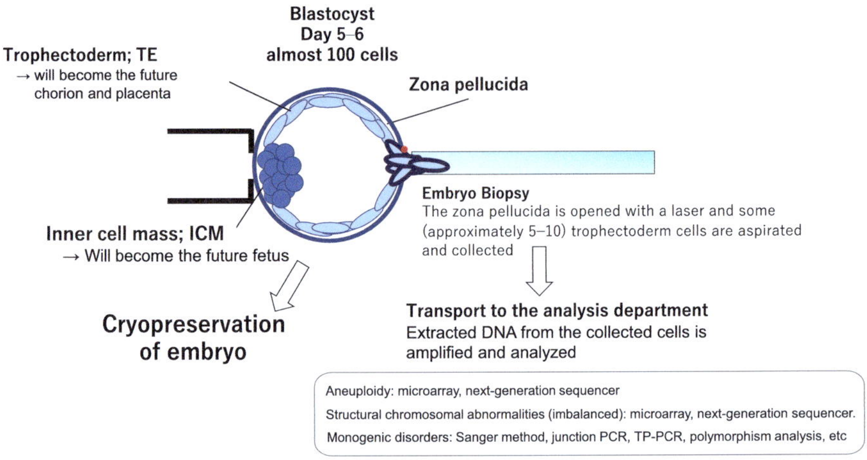

Fig. 7.1 Procedure of preimplantation genetic testing(PGT)

7.2 About PGT-M

Preimplantation genetic testing (PGT) is a technique used in in vitro fertilization and assisted reproductive technology to biopsy a few cells from embryos during in vitro culture and perform tests using chromosomal and genetic analyses. Typically performed during the blastocyst stage on days 5–6 of in vitro culture, a few cells (five to ten cells) are biopsied from the trophectoderm, the outer layer of the embryo that is distant from the inner cell mass (ICM), which will become the fetus. After amplifying the genomic DNA extracted from this cell mass, the desired genetic analysis is performed (Fig. 7.1).

When targeting single-gene disorders, the procedure is referred to as PGT for monogenic disorders (PGT-M), which aims to analyze the presence of pathogenic variants causing the disorder. The analysis methods for PGT-M typically include a "direct approach" of detecting the pathogenic variant and an "indirect approach" using polymorphic markers to estimate the presence of the disorder based on the transmission of the pathogenic allele/wild-type allele to the embryo.

7.3 History of PGT-M in Japan

Following the implementation of the first case of PGT-M targeting X-linked disorders in the UK in 1990, the Japan Society of Obstetrics and Gynecology (JSOG) released the "Statement on Preimplantation Diagnosis" in 1998 [1]. This statement did not explicitly specify the severity interpretation of hereditary diseases that appeared appropriate for PGT-M. At the time of its release, many domestic patient groups with hereditary diseases primarily opposed the implementation of PGT-M, and discussions between these patient groups and JSOG were subsequently held to determine under what circumstances the PGT-M would be permissible. As a result, at that time, it was agreed upon as a criterion appropriate for "genetic disorder that manifest in infancy or childhood death before adulthood due to the lack of effective treatment, or diseases that, even if not fatal, severely impair daily life, such as requiring mechanical ventilation for life support" as the standard, and it was decided to be reviewed and assessed by individual cases not by the disease name. Therefore, as of February 2024, PGT-M has not been performed for HBOC. However, in 2018, approximately 20 years after this decision, a patient couple with a pathogenic variant of hereditary cancer that did not meet the aforementioned severity criteria submitted an application to JSOG, which led to a revision of the statement in January 2022 [2, 3]. In the new statement, considering changes in the interpretation of the "severity of the disease" over time, a neutral review process was established, incorporating the opinions of primary physicians and their respective specialty societies who are responsible for diagnosing and treating patients with relevant hereditary diseases, besides JSOG (obstetrician–gynecologists). This process aims to comprehensively review the applications, considering not only medical judgments but also applicants' living backgrounds and positions, and leaves room for further discussion on the appropriateness of PGT-M for late-onset hereditary diseases such as HBOC.

7.4 Initiatives and Position of JSOG on PGT-M in Japan

According to the Maternal Health Act, compared to PGT, prenatal genetic testing (PNT), a genetic test conducted "after" pregnancy is confirmed, may lead to the decision of pregnancy termination owing to the psychological and economic burden faced by the mother if the pregnancy is continued. Conversely, PGT-M involves testing embryos "before" implantation, leading to less burden on the mother and is considered bioethically "better." Although PNT decisions are made by each couple based on "individual" circumstances, such as their life stage and family planning, JSOG's approval of PGT-M may be perceived, as the "academic organization" does not encourage babies to be born with certain hereditary diseases. Discriminatory or negative effects on people with the hereditary diseases due to the PGT-M approval from JSOG are a major concern. Therefore, JSOG has been cautious with its approach to PGT-M arguments over the past 20 years to avoid being perceived as promoting eugenics. Regarding PGT-M, perspectives not only from couples who are carriers of pathogenic variants for hereditary diseases on PGT-M but also from patients and families living with the diseases, as well as from common people living in society without a specified connection to such hereditary diseases, must be considered. To foster understanding about opinions in society and that perceptions on PGT-M vary from person to person, JSOG has publicly released informative videos titled, "Consideration for Preimplantation Genetic Testing for Couples (Part 1) (Part 2)" in its website to promote further understanding through educational activities [5].

In light of the revision of its statement on PGT-M, JSOG has expressed its fundamental stance on considering the bioethics of reproductive and perinatal medicine both domestically and internationally to clarify its position for future actions as a society [4]. This includes expressing the hope for a tolerant society where consideration and respect are given to individuals with different perspectives and positions. Moreover, all JSOG members, while maintaining this hope, can tolerate complicated situations without clear answers, i.e., negative capability, and respect and implement decisions made while considering opposing opinions (disagree and commit) to ensure that all citizens lead healthy lives as physicians.

7.5 Establishment of a Public Platform in Japan

Currently, no international guidelines suggest recommendations for PGT-M targeting HBOC, and various discussions on this theme are ongoing. PGT-M relates to both the concept of "normalization," which aims for a society where people with and without disabilities support each other and live lively and rich lives in their communities, and the concept of "sexual and reproductive health/rights (SRHR)," which refer to the rights of individuals to make informed decisions about their sexual and reproductive health, free from discrimination, coercion, and violence, for example, whether to have children and when and how many children to have in their lives considering their sexual and reproductive well-being. Concerns have been raised about the current situation where a single professional organization, JSOG, makes decisions on the appropriateness of PGT-M. JSOG requests the government for the establishment of a "public platform for deliberating, supervising, and operating reproductive bioethics."

References

1. Japan Society of Obstetrics and Gynecology. Statement on "Pre-implantation diagnosis". J Japan Soc Obst Gynecol. 1999;51(1):16–43. (in Japanese)
2. Japan Society of Obstetrics and Gynecology. Statements and regulations on ethics: statement on "Pre-implantation genetic testing for serious genetic diseases". 2022a. (in Japanese). https://www.jsog.or.jp/modules/statement/index.php?content_id=3.

3. Japan Society of Obstetrics and Gynecology. Fundamental stance of the Japan Society of Obstetrics and Gynecology on considering ethics related to reproductive and perinatal medicine. 2022b. (in Japanese). https://www.jsog.or.jp/activity/rinri/202203_rinri_kihon.pdf.
4. Japan Society of Obstetrics and Gynecology. Recommendations by the Japan Academy (Establishment of a Public Platform for Proper Operation of Pre-implantation Genetic Testing (PGT) with Ethical Challenges—Focusing on Pre-implantation Genetic Testing (PGT-M) for Hereditary Diseases). 2023. (in Japanese). https://www.jsog.or.jp/modules/committee/index.php?content_id=311.
5. Japan Society of Obstetrics and Gynecology. Public video: Pre-implantation Genetic Testing for Serious Genetic Diseases (PGT-M). n.d.. (in Japanese). https://www.jsog.or.jp/modules/committee/index.php?content_id=257
6. Sasaki A, Takae M, Nishigaki, M. Genetic counseling regarding reproduction: how should it be addressed? HBOC clinical guidelines 2021 edition P78. 2021. (in Japanese).

Chapter 8
HBOC and PGT-M: Social and Ethical Issues and History Regarding PGT-M in Japan

Azumi Tsuge

8.1 Introduction

Since the late 1990s in Japan, diverse opinions have been expressed regarding both preimplantation genetic testing for monogenic disease (hereinafter referred to as PGT-M) and prenatal testing. These opinions have undergone a number of shifts according to advances in genetic testing technologies, medical care, and changes in social welfare policies.

First, I present the Japanese concept of "hereditary disease" and a brief history of eugenics as important background of the concept. Then I discuss PGT-M for hereditary breast and ovarian cancer syndrome (HBOC).

Hasegawa and Igarashi reported the results of their survey asking respondents about their concept of the word of "Iden-byo" (hereditary diseases). The respondents included medical school students (67), nursing school students and nurses (127), childcare students (including teachers) (220), and nutrition students (10) [1]. The respondents were mostly female whose ages ranged from 19 to 85. Results show that most the common response was "fear," followed by pity/sympathy ("pitiful," "painful"), disgust/avoidance ("unpleasant feeling," "don't want to inherit," "troublesome when getting married"), anxiety/worry ("anxious," "worried until childbirth"), and pessimism/regret ("sad", "regrettable"), in that order. Compared to the nursing and medical groups, the childcare and general groups had a higher association rate of fear.

Considering the concepts of reproduction and genetics in Japan, it is vital to remember the human rights violations brought about by the Eugenic Protection Law (1948–1996). Following WWII, Japan's new constitution was characterized by the abandonment of imperialism and the military forces, the abolition of the

A. Tsuge (✉)
Faculty of Sociology, Meiji Gakuin University, Minato, Tokyo, Japan
e-mail: tsuge@soc.meijigakuin.ac.jp

T. Ohta et al. (eds.), *Practical Guide to Hereditary Breast and Ovarian Cancer III*, https://doi.org/10.1007/978-981-96-6779-6_8

old-fashioned patriarchal system, the elimination of social classes, gender inequality, and so on. Replacing the National Eugenic Law of 1940, the Eugenic Protection Law was enacted in 1948 just after with the new constitution. Under the patriarchal system of the old constitution, genetic disorders had been perceived as a stigma or disgrace of the family, ignorant of much of the science of heredity. In effect, the new law promoted prejudice against those suffering from specific diseases or disabilities and strengthened eugenic ideas as a way to prevent "reverse selection of the population" due to social turmoil and population explosion in spite of the social policies of the new constitution. As a result, it became national policy to impose forced sterilizations and abortions on those with certain genetic characteristics, bringing about serious effects on their lives and family planning. Takashi Yokoyama states that "ultimately, genetic counseling is clearly in the lineage of voluntary eugenic marriage consultation that has continued since the introduction of eugenics and continues to influence the current understanding of human genetics." [2]

Looking back to the late 1960s and 1980s, advocate groups for radical disability rights such as the "*Aoi Shiba no Kai*" (the Green Grass Association) began a movement to abolish the Eugenic Protection Law, which, they claimed, violated human reproductive rights, and brought about a fierce opposition movement against the introduction of amniocentesis as tool for prenatal diagnosis.

In 1981, efforts for normalization finally began in Japan with the International Year of Disabled Persons evidenced by the rise of a number of advocacy groups. In 1986, the Disabled Peoples' International (DPI) Japan Council was established. This Japanese affiliate of the international organization focused on the rights of persons with disabilities and the abolition of the Eugenic Protection Law. The DPI Women's Network was also established, with a focus on promoting the independence of women with disabilities as well as the aims of DPI Japan. The DPI Japan Council was also founded in the same vein as the ideology of the *Aoi Shiba no Kai*.

The period 1994–95 saw the introduction of the concept of Reproductive Health/Rights. In one event, a female Japanese member of the DPI Women's Network participating in the NGO conference of the International Conference for Population and Development (ICPD) in Cairo 1994 condemned the Eugenic Protection Law for violating the reproductive rights of the disabled. Garnering both Japanese and international attention, this condemnation led to the Eugenic Protection Law undergoing a major review with many organizations and groups working toward its repeal.

The Eugenic Protection Law was finally revised in 1996, with the problematic "eugenic thought" deleted from its text and the law renamed the "Maternal Protection Law." Despite these landmark revisions, no efforts had been made for apologies, compensation, or restoration of human rights for those who were subjected to forced sterilizations or abortions under the Eugenic Protection Law until one victim's diligent efforts and her advocacy enabled many other victims to file victims lawsuits, gain support for those lawsuits, and finally achieve justice with the landmark Supreme Court ruling on their side.

In July 2024, the Supreme Court ruled that the Eugenic Protection Law had been unconstitutional since its enactment, that the failure of the National Diet to abolish this law for 48 years was a dereliction of duty by the Diet members, and that the country should apologize and compensate those who were subjected to sterilization surgeries or abortions under this law. Finally, the prime minister, Kishida Fumio, apologized to victims of sterilizations and abortions due to the Eugenic Protection Law.

8.2 The Logic Behind the Pros and Cons of PGT-M Since the 1990s

As shown above, Japanese history on the law and concept of hereditary disease has influenced the discussion on the introduction and clinical application of preimplantation diagnosis since the 1990s. The criticisms of PGT-M as well as prenatal testing were not due to the resistance to abortion, or to the discarding of fertilized eggs/embryos, such as that found in the Christian cultural sphere but rather to the deep moral question of "Is it better for people with severe hereditary disease not to be born?" and the criticism that "It is eugenics and should not be done" to confirm the absence of the disease or its genes before birth.

Therefore, the application of PGT-M has been controversial, and opinions differ depending on the position and experience of the patients with the disease, their parents, and those who are about to have children. There are differences in opinions on whether to agree/disagree with the existence of the test, whether to desire or not desire the detailed genetic information provided by the test, and whether to even take the test or not.

The following points have been raised as advantages of applying PGT-M worldwide:

1. Prevent the birth of children with specific genetic diseases.
2. Prevent abortions following prenatal testing.
3. Enable "the birth of savior siblings" who can act as donors for cord blood or bone marrow transplantation to save a sick sibling.
4. Enable sex selection.
5. Allocate more generous medical and social welfare resources who are born with diseases.

On the other hand, the critical or passive opinions include

1. Opposition to the discarding of embryos after genetic screening.
2. Even when preventing the inheritance of genetic diseases, embryo selection denies the existence of people with that disease/disability, thus leading to eugenics/discrimination.
3. The scope of genetic testing will continue to expand, leading to a slippery slope toward eugenics.
4. Physical burden on women by the use of in vitro fertilization and embryo transfer for the test.
5. The success rate of embryo transfer after PGT-M is not high.

6. PGT-M may negatively impact the embryo due to the accompanying embryo biopsy.
7. Patients with the same genetic variant have differences in the severity of their symptoms. Preimplantation diagnosis can only diagnose the presence of the genetic variant, not the severity of the disease.

Among these issues, the most critical discussions in Japan often revolve around the second and third points.

The "*Yusei Shiso wo tou Network*" (Network of Questioning Eugenic Thought), which was at the center of the opposition movement to preimplantation diagnosis in the 1990s and 2000s, argued that the degree of severity "cannot be decided by anyone." This is difficult for medical doctors to understand due to the discrepancy between what doctors think is "good" and how some patients with hereditary diseases believe that they are happy to be born.

In 1995, the University of Kagoshima applied to the Institution Research Ethics Board for clinical application of genetic diagnosis by embryo biopsy. Protests were immediately organized by disability groups, patient groups (such as the Hemophilia Association), and citizen groups that later led to the formation of the *Yusei Shiso wo tou Network.*

Although the Japan Society of Obstetrics and Gynecology (hereinafter JSOG) published the Guidelines for Prenatal Genetic Diagnosis (hereinafter PGD) in 1997, the *Yusei Shiso wo tou Network* sent questions about and criticisms of the JSOG Guidelines, causing JSOG to postpone enforcing the guidelines. After holding two public symposia on PGD, JSOG announced the revised guidelines in 1998. They emphasized that the new guidelines allowed for only severe diseases to undergo PGD, not according to specific diseases, which would recall the nightmares of the Eugenic Protection Law but examining each request by case by case. However, not only *the Yusei Shiso wo tou Network* but also the Japan Muscular Dystrophy Association sent objection letters to JSOG to promote clinical research on PGD. In the end, JSOG did not allow the University of Kagoshima to proceed with their case but did allow Keio University to conduct a preimplantation diagnosis for a case of Duchenne muscular dystrophy in 2004.

8.3 Different Positions and Experiences, and Diverse Opinions Surrounding PGT-M

Here I list the pros and cons of PGD according to my field notes from the Patient/Family Discussion on Genetic Diagnosis hosted by the Japan Muscular Dystrophy Association in Tokyo on May 18, 1996. I encountered a number of diverse opinions and perspectives. I briefly summarize some of these opinions from Muscular Dystrophy (MD) patients, their relatives, and medical doctors.

There were ten panelists: three of them (A, C, D) were young men with MD; the other four were parents of MD patients, while the other three were medical doctors concerned with MD disease.

A, C, and D had different opinions and attitudes about prenatal diagnosis and PGD.

A: I am pro prenatal diagnosis. I believe that parents should not have children if they cannot be responsible for rearing their children… I am glad I was born. I have had some hard times, but I know I must come to terms with it and live with it.

C: I believe I am neither unhappy nor unlucky. It's regrettable if people can easily reject a fetus (with the MD gene), and then the fetus cannot be born because of prenatal diagnosis. The mothers of healthy children say "sorry" to us. However, I wonder if they were assuming that parents raising children with MD are sorry or just pitiful.

D: Although I desire to have my MD be treated, I am concerned about the new genetic therapy. I am not against PGD for MD; however, I think that we don't have enough information about PGD… I think patients really want to have children, even if they have MD, because they feel prenatal diagnosis leads to self-denial.

For those who affirm the "life" of those currently living and trying to improve their living conditions, they feel that they are being denied as a person or as a family member/companion if they agree to prenatal diagnosis or PGD. They are actually being prevented from having a child with MD.

They also ask this question: Isn't it those with the target disease of the prenatal diagnosis that shouldn't be born? One parent (mother) expressed their choice of not wanting to use genetic diagnosis so that she had another child with MD after her first son with MD passed away at 15 years old. She said she and her husband are happy to raise the child with MD as well as others without MD. Another parent (mother) whose two sons passed away from MD explained that her daughter decided not to have a carrier test before getting married in agreement with her partner.

Nobuko Mikata, who lives on her own with part-time carers because of her disease, Spinal Muscular Atrophy (SMA), was shocked by JSOG's approval of the clinical test preimplantation diagnosis in 2004. Therefore, she established the "*Shinkeikin Shikkan Network*" (Neuromuscular Disease Network) with her fellow patients. She explained the reasons for opposing prenatal diagnosis and preimplantation diagnosis as follows:

> When I was in my 20s, in the national nursing home, I saw the families of deceased MD patients come to the daycare for medical examinations years later, and I felt an indescribable anxiety. "Is it so distasteful that a child with muscular dystrophy be born?" I thought, feeling distressed [3].

In 2004, JSOG established the medical indications for parents to use PGT-M if their child would have significant impairments in daily life before reaching adulthood or life-threatening conditions. JSOG's new guidelines for PGT-M were reformed in 2022, which loosened the medical indications because some parents wanted to use

PGT-M despite the diseases not being life-threatening but still requiring invasive treatments.

However, the severity of a given disease can change greatly depending on the degree of medical support, living environment, care/welfare resources, human relationships, etc. Therefore, there is a question how we can say that "it is better not to be born" at the stage of a fertilized egg.

It is also important to consider the logic of "it's good even if it's not cured," which is often heard from the affected parties. Thus, there is a need to listen to the claims of "wanting to live a more human life (with dignity)" rather than the claims for a simple desire for a cure. Within the disability movement, there is a common philosophy that questions the medical approach that emphasizes a cure over improving quality of life.

At the same time, there exists a social value that demands a cure, separate from the patient's own desire to be cured. For those who affirm the "life" of those with incurable diseases or disabilities and try to improve their living conditions in that state, they also feel that patients and their family members and companions are being denied their personal rights. Listening to a mother expressing a strong desire not to pass on the disease gene to her child at the JSOG "PGT-M Ethics Committee," I recalled the scene where the Wexler sisters confronted their parents, saying "why did you have a child?" [4] and thought about the cruelty of hereditary diseases and gender issues.

8.4 Thoughts on the Social and Ethical Issues on Genetic Testing and PGT-M Regarding Hereditary Breast and Ovarian Cancer (HBOC)

Finally, I discuss genetic testing for BRCA1 and/or the BRCA2 variant along with the right to know and the right not to know. I then describe the ethical and social issues regarding PGT-M on HBOC.

Considering the choice of genetic testing, I suggest that one has the right to know one's genetic status as well as the right not to know it. An excellent book to consider the right not to know your genetic status is Alice Wexler's, *Mapping Fate: A Memoir of Family, Risk, and Genetic Research: A Family Confronting Genetic Diagnosis* (1996 = 2003). After their mother suffered from Huntington's disease, once considered incurable, the family poured their effort into researching the disease. Alice Wexler wrote that this disease had been the target of eugenics in the past, and still imposes a heavy burden on people. She wanted to record the recent history of this disease being researched enthusiastically and explored the social and emotional significance of this disease. Once the gene variant of the disease was detected, the genetic test became available but not treatment. The sisters each decided not to undergo genetic testing for Huntington's disease. Their reasons were varied; however, readers can understand their decision from the book.

Nowadays, several issues are discussed about genetic carrier testing as follows:

A positive test result can prepare carriers for early detection and early treatment for future health risks. However, they may experience anxiety and stress. They are likely to have concerns about discrimination by employers or insurance companies if their health risks are leaked. The possibility of discrimination based on the results of genetic testing, particularly in relation to marriage and having children, increases. Furthermore, not informing a marriage partner of being a carrier of a hereditary disease may raise moral issues. On the other hand, if a carrier is unaware of the carrier risks before marriage, not informing a partner is not necessarily a moral issue. This quandary remains a difficult issue in Japan where the concept of an old-fashioned family system is alive and well, and discrimination remains strong toward hereditary diseases as described above.

Parents always want the best for their children's health. Some parents may seek to use PGT-M even, or especially, when they are expecting a healthy baby. These hopes and desires are certainly understandable, but the technology still comes with some risks and pointed critiques by the opponents of PGT-M.

8.5 Conclusion

When accepting genetic testing and expanding its applications, the lessons shown in the case of the Eugenic Protection Law must be remembered. Many Japanese are unaware that this law persisted for half a century, allowing twenty thousand sterilizations or abortions to be carried out for reasons of mental, intellectual, and physical disabilities, and poverty.

PGT-M can be seen as a form of modern eugenics, where certain genetic conditions are selected, and allowing modern eugenics to potentially devalue human lives with those conditions. There are also concerns that PGT-M could lead to discrimination against people with hereditary disease or genetic conditions, resulting in stressful and emotionally challenging conditions for prospective parents, especially those with personal experience of genetic conditions.

Many in the disability community see PGT-M as a threat, as it implies that certain lives are not worth living and thus should be prevented. There are also concerns that the use of PGT-M could lead to a slippery slope to go beyond "severe" conditions to include less severe or even nonmedical traits, ultimately resulting in a decline in social support and resources for certain disabled. There are questions about who should decide which genetic conditions are "severe" to warrant PGT-M. It is important to respect the feelings of those who wish to have children through PGT-M for various reasons. At the same time, we should understand the background behind the desire of "wanting to undergo testing" and not seek solutions solely through medicine.

Overall, the use of PGT-M raises complex ethical and social issues that require careful consideration and ongoing dialogue between medical professionals, policy-makers, disability advocates, and the broader public.

All people including medical professionals should also contribute to efforts for social solutions that address issues beyond medical capabilities. I believe that the choice to undergo testing to prevent the birth of children with specific genetic disorders for various reasons should be respected. However, people who undergo testing may bear a psychological burden regardless of whether they choose to have children or not. Furthermore, we must be cautious about creating a society that makes those who choose not to undergo testing feel solely responsible for their decision.

Enacting a law against genetic discrimination is one way of doing so. However, discrimination can still be found daily, much of which is difficult to regulate by law. I thus emphasize that our aim should be instead to maintain a society in which those born with "severe" hereditary disease can say that they are happy to have been born. We must continue efforts to realize a society in which parents and others do not feel pity for those born with congenital diseases. That may take time, but history shows that it is possible.

References

1. Hasegawa T, Igarashi T. Popular image of the term 'GeneticDisease'. Tokyo Women's Med Univ J. 1993;63:94–101.
2. Yokoyama T. "Shushozen Shindan no Rekishi to Genzai—Jihatsuteki Yuseigaku no Keifu" (The History and Present of Prenatal Diagnosis: The Genealogy of Voluntary Eugenics). J Japan Soc Health Sci. 2021;87(4):139–60.
3. Mikata N. "Inochi no Senbetsu wo sarerugawa no doshinen" (Concentric circles on the side of the selection of life). In: Action Committee of Yusei Shiso wo Hogusu, *Yusei Shiso wo Hogusu* (Unwind Eugenic Thinking). Kyoto; 2023. p. 16–8.
4. Wexler A. Mapping fate: a memoir of family, risk, and genetic research a family confronting genetic diagnosis. University of California Press; 1996. Muto, Kaori and Nukaga,Yoshio translated into Japanese 2003, *Wexler ke no sentaku*, Shinchosha Publisher, Tokyo, Japan.

Chapter 9
Social Challenges of Preimplantation Genetic Testing for Monogenic Disorders (PGT -M)in HBOC and Medical Professional Recognition

Hiromi Arakawa and Arisa Ueki

Abstract **Background:** Many kinds of hereditary cancers are inherited with a 50% chance of autosomal dominant transmission. In several countries, mainly in Europe and North America, prenatal diagnosis (PND) and preimplantation genetic testing for monogenic disorders (PGT-M) are recognized as reproductive options for individual with hereditary cancers. However, there are no reports of PGT-M for hereditary cancer being performed in Japan at this time, and there are few reports on the awareness of PGT-M among medical professionals specializing in oncology.

Objective: This study aimed to survey the awareness and perspectives regarding reproductive medical technologies, particularly PGT-M, among healthcare professionals affiliated with cancer care facilities. Based on these results, we identified and discussed issues related to the provision of PGT-M information.

Participants and Methods: An Internet-based questionnaire survey was conducted among medical professionals affiliated with the Cancer Institute Hospital Ariake and its affiliated research institute, a specialized cancer care facility.

Results: Of 509 survey participants, 499 consented to participate. Among the respondents, 380 (76%) were aware of PND, 99 (20%) had heard of it, and 20 (4%) had never heard about it. In contrast, 36 (7%) were aware of the PGT-M, and 71 (14%) had heard of it. In response to the question "Do you think there are people diagnosed with hereditary cancer who would like to undergo PGT-M/PND in Japan?" more than 90% of the respondents answered "Yes, I think there are" or "I think there are people who would like to hear an explanation."

Discussion: The discrepancy in awareness of PGT-M and PND among health-cre professionals may stem from varying opportunities to access information. In Japan, the target diseases or conditions for PGT-M are limited, and oncology health-care providers have insufficient opportunities to obtain information. In the future,

H. Arakawa · A. Ueki (✉)
Department of Clinical Genetics Oncology, Cancer Institute Hospital of JFCR, Koto-Ku, Tokyo, Japan
e-mail: arisa.ueki@jfcr.or.jp

T. Ohta et al. (eds.), *Practical Guide to Hereditary Breast and Ovarian Cancer III*, https://doi.org/10.1007/978-981-96-6779-6_9

oncology healthcare professionals will acquire the knowledge necessary to provide information about PGT-M and refer patients to specialists.

Keywords Preimplantation genetic testing for monogenic disorders (PGT-M) · Prenatal diagnosis (PND) · Questionnaire survey · Medical professional recognition · HBOC

9.1 Introduction

Hereditary cancer syndromes predispose individuals to certain cancers due to pathogenic variants in the germline of specific genes. Individuals diagnosed with hereditary cancer syndromes can significantly benefit from appropriate surveillance and medical interventions.

For instance, women diagnosed with hereditary breast and ovarian cancer (HBOC) are at high risk of developing breast and ovarian cancers [1]. Effective strategies are breast surveillance by contrast-enhanced breast magnetic resonance imaging (MRI) or risk-reducing mastectomy [2, 3]. However, there is no effective surveillance for ovarian cancer; therefore, several guidelines recommend risk-reducing salpingo-oophorectomy after childbearing is complete. [2, 3]. Consequently, women of reproductive age with HBOC need to consider their life plans while taking precautions against breast and ovarian cancers. Additionally, the risk of transmitting germline pathogenic variants that cause hereditary cancers to offspring remains a concern and may influence future pregnancies. [4].

If one partner carries a pathogenic variant associated with hereditary cancer, prenatal diagnosis (PND) and preimplantation genetic testing for monogenic disorders (PGT-M) are options to prevent transmission of the pathogenic variant to offspring. PND is performed after conception through chorionic villus sampling or amniocentesis. If PND indicates a genetic condition in the fetus, the couple may decide whether to continue with the pregnancy. In contrast, PGT-M is conducted before conception and involves genetic testing of embryos obtained via in vitro fertilization. Only embryos without the targeted genetic condition are implanted, reducing the likelihood that the couple will have to consider terminating the pregnancy because of a genetic condition.

In several countries, PGT-M is already a clinical option for hereditary cancers. The European Society of Human Reproduction (ESHRE) approved PGT-M in 2003, and the United Kingdom's Human Fertilization and Embryology Authority (HFEA) approved it in 2006 for hereditary cancers with adult-onset and non-100% penetrance, such as HBOC [5, 6]. In Japan, the Japan Society of Obstetrics and Gynecology (JSOG) revised its stance on "Pre-Implantation Genetic Testing for Monogenic (PGT-M) for Serious Genetic Disorders" after careful discussions with genetic experts and stakeholders in 2022 [7]. As of February 2023, there have been no reports of PGT-M for hereditary cancers in Japan. Nonetheless, PGT-M has been increasingly discussed among geneticists, obstetricians, gynecologists, genetic oncologists, and patients with hereditary cancers. There are limited reports in Japan on the awareness and perspectives of cancer careprofessionals regarding genetic and reproductive health, including PGT-M. Therefore, this study surveyed health-carel professionals in a specialized oncology facility to assess their awareness and perspectives about reproductive options such as PGT-M. Based on these results, we aimed to clarify the current situation regarding hereditary cancer and PGT-M among cancer care professionals and discuss future challenges.

9.2 Materials and Methods

We surveyed the awareness and perspectives of healthcare professionals at specialized cancer treatment facilities regarding reproductive options, particularly for PGT-M. Based on the survey results, we identified and discussed issues related to the provision of information on PGT-M and other cancer treatments.

The survey was conducted among healthcare professionals affiliated with the Cancer Institute Hospital of the Japanese Foundation for Cancer Research and its associated research institutes. Physicians and nurses and other healthcare professionals affiliated with the Cancer Institute Hospital and Research Institute were invited to participate via email. The survey response period lasted approximately one month, from November 25, 2022, to December 31, 2022. The surveys were conducted anonymously.

The original questionnaire, administered through Google Forms, assessed knowledge and perspectives on prenatal testing and PGT-M. Consent for participation was obtained prior to completion of the questionnaire.

9.3 Results

- **Participants' Characteristics**
  Of the 509 survey participants, 499 provided consent for participation. Table 9.1 shows the characteristics of all respondents. A total of 117 respondents (24%) were male, and 381 (76%) were female. Among the respondents, 264 (53%) were nurses and 107 (21%) were physicians, accounting for 74% of all respondents. The respondents' ages ranged from their 20s to their 70s. Their experience in the oncology field ranged from less than one year to more than 20 years.
  The survey was sent to all hospital medical staff via an in-house email inviting all "medical professionals." Each participant had a different level of involvement in cancer care, medical knowledge, and interaction with patients and their families.

- **Awareness of healthcare professionals involved in oncology about PND and PGT-M**

Table 9.1 Participant characteristics

Demographic variables	%	$n = 499$
Sex		
Male	23.4	117
Female	76.9	381
Unknown	0.2	1
Professional variables		
Doctor	21.4	107
Nurse	52.9	264
Clinical laboratory technologist	7.0	35
Nursing assistant	3.8	19
Pharmacist	3.6	18
Clinical research coordinator	1.2	6
Medical social worker	1.0	5
Genetic counselor	1.0	5
Others	8.0	40
Presence of children		
Yes	43.1	215
No	56.9	284
Age		
Up to 29 years old	16.8	84
30–39	31.7	158
40–49	29.5	147
50–59	15.4	77
60–69	6.0	30
Over 70 years old	0.6	3
Years of clinical experience in oncology		
Up to 1 y	6.6	33
3 y	11.4	57
5 y	11.2	56
10 y	23.4	117
15 y	18.2	91
20 y	11.2	56
Over 20 years old	17.8	89

All respondents (n = 499) were asked about their awareness of PND and PGT-M; 380 (76%) were aware of PND, 99 (20%) had heard of it, and 20 (4%) were unaware of it. In contrast, only 36 respondents (7%) were aware of PGT-M, 71 (14%) had heard of it, and 392 (79%) were unaware of it. For PGT-M, the total of those who "knew" and "had heard of" it was approximately 21%, indicating a significant discrepancy in awareness between PGT-M and PND (Fig. 9.1a). Among the 107 respondents who "knew" or "had heard" of PGT-M, 25 respondents (23.4%) knew the difference between PGT-M and PND, and 32 respondents (29.9%) had heard of the difference.

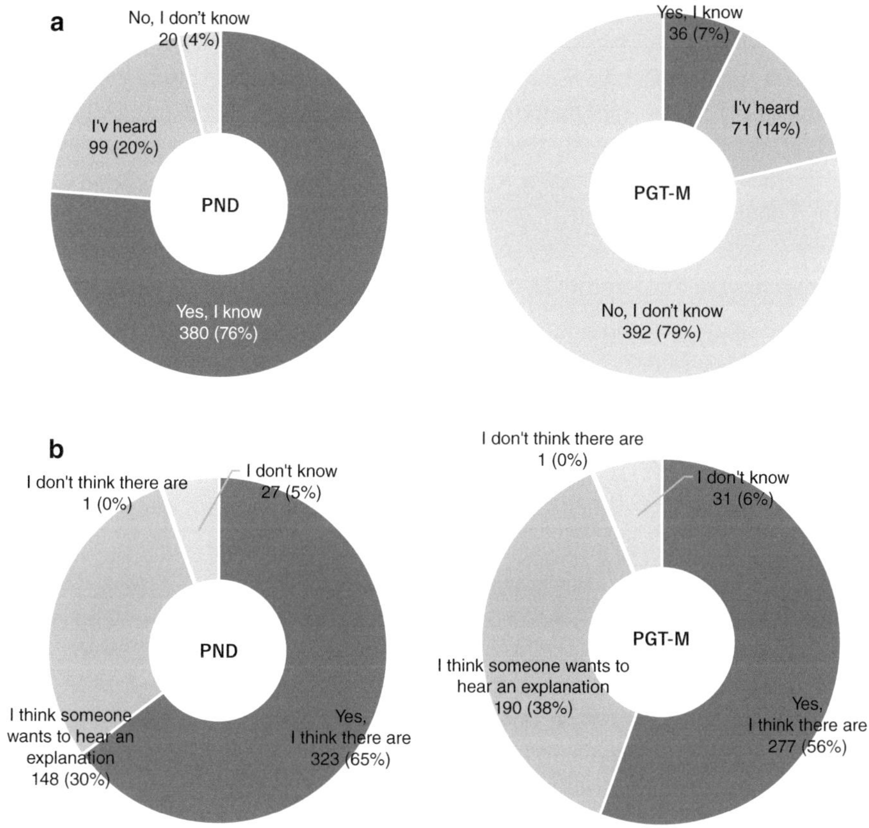

Fig. 9.1 (**a**) Awareness about prenatal diagnosis (PND) and preimplantation genetic testing (PGT-M) monogenic defect (PGT-M). (**b**) Do you think there are individuals who would like to have *PGT-M/PND* for hereditary cancer in Japan?

Although the survey was conducted at a single institution, the awareness of PGT-M among oncology healthcare professionals was insufficient.

- **Needs for PGT-M and PND based on hereditary cancers considered by healthcare professionals at base hospitals for cancer treatment**

If the respondents had insufficient knowledge of PND and PGT-M, a brief description of these procedures for hereditary cancer was added to the questionnaire. After reading the text, the respondents answered questions on PND and PGT-M for hereditary cancer.

In response to the question, "Do you think there are individual diagnosed with hereditary cancer who would like to undergo PGT-M/PND in Japan?" Regarding PGT-M, 277 respondents (56%) answered, "Yes, I think there are" and 190 respondents (38%) answered, "Yes, there are individual who would like to hear an explanation." For PND, 323 (65%) and 148 (30%) respondents, respectively, answered similarly (Fig. 9.1b).

This result suggests that the heathcare professionals of hospitals specializing in cancer may perceive a need for PGT-M for hereditary cancers.

9.4 Discussion

- **Awareness of PND and PGT-M**

In this survey, over 90% of the participants were aware of PND, whereas only 21% were aware of PGT-M. This significant difference in awareness can be attributed to the lack of information and clinical experience with PGT-M among cancer care providers.

The rapid expansion of noninvasive prenatal testing (NIPT) is one reason PND has become widely known in Japan: NIPT screening for trisomy 13, 18, and 21 in fetuses. These chromosomal aneuploidies can occur in any fetus. In Japan, NIPT began in 2013 as a clinical study at a limited number of facilities and quickly expanded because testing was conducted at locations without adequate genetic counseling systems. To address this issue, the expert committee of the Ministry of Health, Labour, and Welfare submitted the "Report of the Expert Committee on NIPT and Other Prenatal Tests" in 2021.

According to this report, it is appropriate to provide information about PND, including NIPT, to pregnant women and their partners in a nondirective manner. This topic has been covered by various media outlets, raising awareness among medical professionals and the general public.

In contrast, PGT-M is limited to cases in which one or both partners carry a genetic variant or chromosomal translocation that may result in serious genetic disorders. Couples wishing to undergo PGT-M in Japan must apply to a review committee for individual cases within the JSOG for approval. If granted, PGT-M is performed. This situation differs significantly from that of PND.

Although it is anticipated that opinions on PGT-M will be revised in 2022 and the range of eligible diseases will be expanded, the implementation of PGT-M for hereditary cancers that develop in adulthood and have incomplete penetrance has not been previously reported.

The reason for the disparity in awareness between the two procedures among healthcare professionals is that prenatal testing is more frequently discussed in academia, society, and the media, regardless of the general public. Hereditary cancers have not been considered an indication for PGT-M, resulting in fewer opportunities for healthcare prpfessionals involved in cancer care to learn about it.

Gietel-Habets et al. reported that specialist knowledge of PGT-M was positively correlated with referral consultations. Although genetic specialists are the primary providers of information on PGT-M, other specialists may serve as initial contacts for consultation with genetic specialists [8].

International guidelines for the treatment and practice of hereditary cancers and statements from academic societies already include recommendations for providing information on PGT-M and other reproductive options [2, 9–11]. It may also be worth considering in Japan to include reproductive information in its guidelines, so that healthcare providers can access it.

- **Needs for PGT-M and PND based on hereditary cancers**

In this study, more than 90% of respondents indicated the need for PGT-M and PND in cases of hereditary cancers. PND involves testing fetal cells obtained after pregnancy through chorionic villus sampling or amniocentesis. If PND reveals a genetic condition in the fetus, the couple may consider and decide whether to continue the pregnancy. In contrast, PGT-M involves the genetic testing of embryos obtained through in vitro fertilization. Only embryos free of the targeted genetic conditions identified by PGT-M are selected for implantation. Couples undergoing PGT-M rarely face the decision to continue the pregnancy due to genetic conditions. This differs significantly from PND, which results in a distinct psychological burden on women.

In 1990, the first preimplantation genetic testing, known as preimplantation genetic diagnosis (PGD), was performed in the United Kingdom on two couples at risk of having children with adrenoleukodystrophy, an X-linked inherited disease [12]. PGT-M is currently indicated for hereditary cancers in Western and Asian countries. According to an ESHRE report, approximately 5% of the PGT-M cases performed in 2018 targeted HBOC [13]. The American Society for Reproductive Medicine considers that PGT-M as a significant scientific advancement for couples at risk of having children with genetic diseases [14], including adult-onset genetic conditions.

Some cancer patients undergo fertility preservation procedures, such as embryo, oocyte, or ovarian freezing, prior to cancer treatment. Patients with hereditary cancers may consider PGT-M as an option if they wish to conceive after cancer treatment. Because PGT-M uses embryos obtained through in vitro fertilization for genetic testing, patients who preserve embryos before cancer treatment may find PGT-M more accessible if they wish to conceive after treatment.

Therefore, it is important to provide consultations and information on techniques such as PGT-M and fertility preservation in the future. Referrals to specialists and specialized facilities capable of providing comprehensive information and performing these procedures should be considered.

Currently, genetic counseling for individuals with hereditary cancers focuses on providing information about increased cancer risk, coping strategies, and implications for family members, as outlined in national and international guidelines. Future pregnancy and childbearing are often discussed, particularly for clients of reproductive age. Even for patients diagnosed with hereditary cancer who have completed their childbearing, access to information about reproductive options, such as PGT-M can provide psychological support whensharing genetic information with their children. Therefore, it is crucial to provide adequate information to all individuals diagnosed with hereditary cancers.

9.5 Limitations of This Survey and Prospects

Approximately half of the medical staff in our institute responded to this survey. Respondents were likely to have a high level of interest in hereditary cancers, PGT-M, or PND. We plan to expand the survey to include genetic specialists, individuals with hereditary cancers, and their families to obtain more comprehensive data on awareness and opinions regarding PGT-M in Japan.

In designing this survey, we considered the possibility that the PGT-M may not be widely known among health professionals providing cancer care. Therefore, a brief explanation was included in the survey. However, the explanatory text may not have adequately addressed the diverse values, beliefs, and ethical perspectives related to PGT-M. Therefore, the findings of this study may not fully capture the perspectives and needs of PGT-M and prenatal testing. Future studies will seek input from individuals diagnosed with hereditary cancers to enhance survey design and interpretation of surveys.

9.6 Conclusion

The survey results indicate that healthcare professionals in oncology facilities recognize the need for PGT-M and PND in patients diagnosed with hereditary cancers. There is an urgent need for healthcare professionals to establish a support system that empowers individuals with hereditary cancer to make informed decisions and live their lives according to their preferences.

Acknowledgments We thank Pfizer Japan Inc. for the Global Medical Grants and Editage (www.editage.jp) for the English language editing.

References

1. Kuchenbaecker KB, et al. Risks of breast, ovarian, and contralateral breast cancer for BRCA1 and BRCA2 mutation carriers. JAMA. 2017;317(23):2402–16.
2. NCCN Clinical practice guidelines in oncology. Genetic/Familial high-risk assessment: breast, ovarian, and pancreatic version 3.2024.
3. Japanese Organization of Hereditary Breast and Ovarian Cancer. Guidelines for diagnosis and treatment of hereditary breast and ovarian cancer. 2021.
4. Chan JL, et al. Reproductive decision-making in women with BRCA1/2 mutations. J Genet Couns. 2017;23(3):594–603.
5. The ESHRE Ethics Task Force. Taskforce 5: preimplantation genetic diagnosis. Hum Reprod. 2003;18(3):649–51.
6. Dyer C. HFEA widens its criteria for preimplantation genetic diagnosis. BMJ. 2006;332(7551):1174.

7. The Japan Society of Obstetrics and Gynecology. The revised opinion Pre-implantation genetic testing for monogenic (PGT-M) for serious genetic disorders. Acta Obstet Gynaecol Jpn. 2023;75(8):796–803. (Original Japanese)
8. Gietel-Habets JJG, et al. Professionals' knowledge, attitude, and referral behaviour of preimplantation genetic diagnosis for hereditary breast and ovarian cancer. Reprod Biomed Online. 2018;36(2):137–44.
9. NCCN Clinical Practice Guidelines in Oncology. Familial High-Risk Assessment: Colorectal Version 2. 2023.
10. Paluch-Shimon S, et al. Prevention and screening in BRCA mutation carriers and other breast/ovarian hereditary cancer syndromes: ESMO Clinical Practice Guidelines for cancer prevention and screening. Ann Oncol. 2016;27(suppl 5):v103–10.
11. Berliner JL, et al. Risk assessment and genetic counseling for hereditary breast and ovarian cancer syndromes-practice resource of the National Society of genetic counselors. J Genet Couns. 2021;30(2):342–60.
12. Handyside AH, et al. Pregnancies from biopsied human preimplantation embryos sexed by Y-specific DNA amplification. Nature. 1990;344(6268):768–70.
13. Spinella F, et al. ESHRE PGT consortium data collection XXI: PGT analyses in 2018. Human Reprod Open. 2023;2023(2)
14. Practice Committee of Society for Assisted Reproductive Technology, et al. Preimplantation genetic testing: a practice committee opinion. Fertil Steril. 2008;90(5 Suppl):S136.

Chapter 10
Statement from a Patient

Makiko Dazai

Abstract We, the hereditary breast and ovarian cancer patient support group "Clavis Arcus" and the genetic disease patient and family support group "Genetic Alliance JP," have been engaged in patient support activities, research projects, and addressing ELSI issues for many years. As medical technology advances, there is a need for a medical care delivery system and social understanding that enables us to obtain accurate information about the medical care available to us and to accept whatever choice is made in an appropriate, safe, and secure manner.

In recent years, while more patients and their blood relatives are undergoing genetic testing as part of their treatment, there have been calls for information about reproductive medicine and PGT-M from parties with hereditary breast and ovarian cancer. Many are considering PGT-M and gathering information.

Conversely, it is necessary to consider the values and thoughts of those who do not wish to undergo PGT-M.

As a hereditary condition, multiple individuals within a family may be affected, and the experiences and perspectives on childbirth can vary based on the severity of the disease and their living environment. I believe that in supporting patients, it is essential to respect each person's thoughts and feelings. Each individual should be consulted after being informed that their perspectives are shaped by their unique way of life and environment and that none of these perspectives can be dismissed. I maintain a neutral position, neither recommending nor discouraging PGT-M. Another important question is how much information needs to be provided in places where people share their thoughts with each other and in individual consulta-

M. Dazai (✉)
Specified Nonprofit Corporation Clavis Arcus, Association of Patients for Hereditary Breast and Ovarian Cancer Syndrome, Tokyo, Japan

Genetic Alliance JP, Shibuya-ku, Tokyo, Japan
e-mail: maki@geneticalliance.jp

T. Ohta et al. (eds.), *Practical Guide to Hereditary Breast and Ovarian Cancer III*, https://doi.org/10.1007/978-981-96-6779-6_10

tions and how to provide support in a way that is not perceived as strongly pointing to the ideas of one side or the other.

For those of us who have developed a disease, it is natural to wish for the health of our own children, and it is common to hope that our descendants born in the future will not develop the same disease or can avoid developing it. I would like to share with you the current situation we have been able to obtain from the support of patients and others in Japan regarding their thoughts on fertility and PGT-M.

Keywords Hereditary breast and ovarian cancer (HBOC) · BRCA1/2 pathologic variant carriers · Unaffected carriers · Risk-reducing mastectomy · Risk-reducing salpingo-oophorectomy (RRSO) · Fertility preservation

10.1 Introduction

As medical technology advances, there is a need for a medical care delivery system and social understanding that enables us to obtain accurate information about the medical care available to us and to "accept" whatever choice is made in an appropriate, safe, and secure manner.

In Japan, fertility issues for cancer patients are becoming well known to many patients and citizens, but PGT-M is not yet a common practice and is only offered to a limited number of patients under certain conditions. However, due to the status of PGT-M in other countries, individual attitudes, and life circumstances, more people with hereditary breast and ovarian cancer are seeking information about PGT-M and actually going abroad for treatment.

Although discussions among medical professionals are progressing, fertility preservation and preimplantation diagnosis, as well as the timing of treatment, pregnancy, and childbirth, and ethical issues are all matters that require serious, real-time decisions for affected patients.

Some people with BRCA1 or BRCA2 genetic mutations avoid pregnancy and childbirth for fear of passing the disease on to their children. Others fear that they will be blamed for choosing life or feel that their existence is being denied.

My answer, derived from many years of supporting people with cancer, is that issues related to pregnancy and childbirth should be decided by the person affected, and no one, not even blood relatives, should be allowed to deny their choice. It is necessary to provide accurate and up-to-date information, as well as medical care and social support that can support and protect those making such decisions, whether they have cancer or not, so that they can make choices in accordance with their environment and wishes.

Although we have discussed this issue with many people with incurable diseases and hereditary tumors, this report is limited to the thoughts of people with hereditary breast and ovarian cancer (HBOC).

10.2 Support Activities to Deepen Understanding of Hereditary Cancer

There are many individuals who feel that the diagnosis of hereditary cancer has overshadowed the pain of developing cancer itself, and if they are parents, they often blame themselves. Additionally, there are important considerations for those diagnosed with HBOC before deciding to forgo pregnancy and childbirth due to the hereditary nature of the disease.

By deepening their understanding of heredity, they will learn the importance of knowing their genetic makeup and the mechanisms of cancer development. The number of individuals who become aware of health management not only for themselves but also for their families continues to increase year by year. In Japan, genetics is often viewed negatively, but with the support of medical professionals and certified genetic counselors, we are working to create many seminars and learning opportunities to help people realize the value of genetics. We believe that with equal and accurate information, individuals need time to think and organize the information with their partners.

We are increasingly discussing how having a child with the possibility of HBOC is not necessarily negative, and that even without the genetic mutation, cancer cannot be completely avoided.

10.3 Will PGT-M Be a Form of Preventative Medicine, Like Risk-Reducing Surgery?

We, the affected individuals, can undergo risk-reducing mastectomy or risk-reducing salpingo-oophorectomy by knowing our genetic status. Insurance coverage is limited to those with HBOC who have developed cancer, but it is possible for those who have not developed cancer to undergo risk-reducing surgery as a medical treatment if they pay for it themselves.

In the past, many of us have experienced times when even wanting risk-reducing surgery as a preventive measure was not understood and was condemned. Only recently it has come to be understood as a preventive medical treatment to reduce risk, prevent cancer, and save lives. Today, it is not accepted by all of the public, and negative views remain both in the general public and among medical professionals. Additionally, some HBOC patients do not want risk-reducing surgery.

As HBOC treatment has become routine and risk-reducing surgery has become equally available as medical care for eligible patients, there is now more information and support for decision-making about how to incorporate preventive medical treatment into one's lifestyle. The creation of an environment in which it is easy to consult with medical professionals has led to a reduction in the psychological burden for us, the affected individuals.

Reasons for not wanting risk-reducing surgery include the patient not being old enough to undergo the procedure, wanting to have a baby between treatments or after settling down post-treatment, concerns about their relationship with their partner (e.g., the impact on their sex life), and the fear that it will undermine their value as a woman. These concerns have been frequently raised in our peer support services.

There are many people who cannot make the decision to have risk-reducing surgery even though they know it will help them avoid developing cancer. No matter how scared they are of getting cancer, they still cannot make the decision.

No matter what choice is made, there is rarely any denial of the other party. It is important to respect and support each other's ideas and values in accordance with their respective lifestyles.

It is conceivable that as medical technology advances in the future, the number of people who wish to have PGT-M among HBOC individuals will increase. Therefore, we should provide accurate and unbiased information and develop a system so that it can be provided safely, securely, and at a reasonable cost throughout the country. Even with a medical care system in place, as with risk-reducing surgery, not everyone will want to undergo it. However, we believe that the psychological and financial burden of seeking treatment abroad when the technology is available is immeasurable.

Genetic preimplantation diagnosis may be the ultimate preventive medicine, but the time may not be far off when it will be incorporated into routine medical care as one of the ways to reduce risk.

10.4 Comments Actually Received from HBOC Patients

Here are some comments actually received from HBOC patients:

(a) I found out I had HBOC after my pregnancy and delivery. If I had known before, I might have been more worried about having a child. However, I do not want HBOC to be a target disease for preimplantation diagnosis.

(b) If I had not been diagnosed with HBOC, I would have wanted to have a baby. I feel that I cannot give up my wish to have a baby, and I have had the opportunity to talk to the people involved, but I have not been able to make a decision. It is hard to think that I might have a hard time if my constitution is inherited and my child develops cancer at a young age. I plan to have an RRSO when I reach the recommended age of 35, so childbirth may be difficult. I hope that PGT-M will be available like in other countries, so that even if I am found to have HBOC in the future (even with preimplantation diagnosis, it is not 100% genetic), I will be able to give birth with peace of mind.

(c) I hope that the ethical aspects of PGT-M will be discussed thoroughly, because it could be the "selection of life" as it is often called. It is very sad to think that we might not have existed in this day and age. I cannot get over the fact that we are so afraid of "discrimination" that we might as well be "sorting" lives.

(d) If the risks are known at the fertilized egg stage, there may be a choice not to have a baby. If medicine can go that far, does not that mean it is okay to use it? Even if there is a one in two chance, I would want to terminate if I can avoid it. I would not hesitate to use PGT-M if I would rather have my children and grandchildren carry the burden and fear as they grow up.

(e) I feel very conflicted. I feel like I am in denial: What will happen after I eliminate all the HBOCs and other genetic mutations? Will I really be happy?

(f) I already knew about PGT-M, so I proactively asked my own doctors and genetic counselors. I think it is an unlikely medical treatment for those of us who have developed "cancer" because there is not enough information and the application and process is time-consuming. I was uncomfortable with the negative attitude of the medical staff when I mentioned the possibility.

(g) Even if I am able to preserve my fertility, I have fear and anxiety that I may have a child who is genetically at risk, even if she has cancer. I don't know where to talk about these feelings. I would like to know where to ask about medical care and government services.

(h) Many of my family members, including my mother, sisters, and aunt, have suffered and died from cancer. After watching them die since I was a child, when I developed cancer, all I could think about was death, and I am still afraid of recurrence or metastasis. I got married before I had genetic testing, but I was afraid to have children because I was tested and diagnosed positive before having children. Every time I remember the end of my family's life, I feel pain in my heart, but I do not want my children to have the same feelings. They say everyone is at risk of getting cancer, but I don't think everyone goes through such a painful experience. I made this decision after discussing it with my husband. If PGT-M will reduce the number of people who will suffer the same sadness in the future, I do not think I can deny that there are people who want to have PGT-M.

(i) I would rather have a medical treatment called PGT-M than give up pregnancy and childbirth for fear of having a genetic mutation.

(j) Many individuals want to avoid having children with mutations in the BRCA1 and BRCA2 genes but are concerned about how they will be perceived socially and ethically. However, the quantity and quality of information provided in Japan is also increasingly mentioned by many individuals. Because the current situation is that even if there are applicants in Japan, the applications and the system itself are not yet in place, and because it is difficult to determine which individual's thoughts are the same, I think the time has come to listen broadly to the voices of many individuals and to think about PGT-M.

10.5 Genetic Medicine Is Medicine of Hope for the Future

Many people have had to forgo pregnancy and childbirth due to illness, even if they do not have HBOC. While I personally believe that a childless lifestyle is not inherently negative, I have observed many patients who feel pressured or blame themselves for the societal emphasis on having healthy and physically satisfying offspring. I believe that medical care, environment, and systems should be provided to support the precious desire to have children and that PGT-M should be equally available to those who wish to have children and those who do not.

Rather than judging the value of a person based on their genetic makeup, the ideal that should be realized, as felt through the support of the affected individuals, is to create a world in which everyone can live comfortably and build a society in which people can respect each other. Right now, medical technology has not yet caught up with measures and shared ideas on social and ethical issues. Again, it will be indispensable in the future that medical care, information, and support are appropriately provided to individuals with HBOC who wish to have PGT-M. Medical technology will continue to evolve and advance day by day, and we have high hopes for measures in genetic medicine to avoid losing one's life to cancer.

10.6 About "Clavis Arcus"

Clavis Arcus is the first and only patient association supporting *BRCA1* and *BRCA2* pathogenic variant carriers and their families in Japan. The organization was established in 2014 and certified as a nonprofit organization by the Tokyo Metropolitan Government in 2015. The organization aims to provide a gathering space for the members to support each other and deepen knowledge and understanding of hereditary tumors. There are 195 members among Japan, and it has a branch in Pennsylvania, USA.

Their organization provides consultations by phone, e-mail, web meeting and in person, as well as holding patients' gatherings. We started the "Institute of Genetic Studies" for further understanding of hereditary cancers and education for peer supporter and hold Learning about Genetics for Families seminars annually.

In addition to providing consultations via phone, email, web conferencing, and in-person meetings, our organization hosts patient exchange meetings. When Clavis Arcus was founded, citizens, patients, patient families, and healthcare professionals wanted to improve understanding of hereditary tumor syndromes, cultivate peer supporters, and establish a place where patients and families could gather and learn together. To convey patients' perspectives to healthcare providers and ensure that everyone could access accurate information through interaction and learning, regardless of location, we created a team within the patient organization called the Institute of "Genetics Study (IGS)" to plan, support, and operate initiatives. Since then, we have held seminars open to anyone. However, the number of facilities willing to provide venues has decreased since the onset of the pandemic, making it difficult to operate as planned. Nevertheless, we intend to continue developing initiatives that empower citizens and patients.

Since 2018, with the cooperation of healthcare professionals nationwide (primarily medical institutions and genetic counselors), we have continuously held photo panel exhibitions across Japan. This exhibition combines photographs and letters from hereditary cancer patients themselves and their families. The panels display the patients' own photographs alongside letters from their families, reaching HBOC patient peers, healthcare professionals, and citizens nationwide. We consider this activity, which conveys patients' voices, to be important and continue to hold the exhibitions. New event information will be posted here (https://www.clavisarcus.com).

10.7 About "Genetic Alliance JP"

Genetic Alliance JP, established through the collaboration and cooperation of patients with hereditary diseases, their families, and related organizations, aims to promote and disseminate appropriate genomic medicine through mutual support, awareness activities, policy advocacy, research activities, and improvements in medical and welfare services. It also works to resolve the social challenges faced by patients with hereditary cancers. To date, 14 organizations related to genomic medicine have joined this alliance. It has also tackled key issues, such as policy advocacy related to the Act on Promotion of Genomic Medicine. Collaborating with organizations focused on hereditary tumor syndromes and intractable diseases, it conducts thorough evaluations from a position directly involved in treatments like PGT-M. It contributes to building systems that support personalized medicine tailored to each individual (https://www.geneticalliance.jp)**.

Part IV
JOHBOC Registration

Chapter 11
Updates to the Registration Data of the Japanese Organization of Hereditary Breast and Ovarian Cancers: Summary for 2022

Mayuko Inuzuka, Takanori Ishida, and Seigo Nakamura

Abstract In recent years, insurance coverage of *BRCA1/2* genetic testing has been expanding in Japan. As one of its projects, the Japanese organization of hereditary breast and ovarian cancer (JOHBOC) conducts a registry of hereditary breast and ovarian cancer (HBOC) for families. A database for HBOC is being established with the aim of describing the clinical and genetic characteristics and linking this to standard treatment by improving the medical treatment environment for the concerned patients and their inclusion in guidelines, and participation is being solicited from medical facilities throughout Japan. This chapter reports a summary of the 2022 data. A total of 134 facilities nationwide participated in this registration project. The enrollment of *BRCA1/2* pathogenic variant carriers was 3610. More than 10% of these were unaffected *BRCA1/2* pathogenic variant carriers. Furthermore, 439 patients undergoing risk-reducing mastectomy (RRM) and 831 patients undergoing risk-reducing salpingo-oophorectomy (RRSO) were enrolled. Since April 2020, surveillance, RRM, and RRSO for HBOC patients with a history of breast or ovarian cancer have been covered by insurance in Japan. Two years have passed since then, and the actual situation of HBOC care in Japan has gradually become clearer. However, HBOC care is not yet covered by insurance for unaffected *BRCA1/2* patho-

M. Inuzuka (✉)
Department of Genetic Counseling, Showa University Graduate School of Health Sciences, Tokyo, Japan

Department of Breast Surgical Oncology, Showa University School of Medicine, Tokyo, Japan
e-mail: inuzuka-m@cnt.showa-u.ac.jp

T. Ishida
Department of Breast and Endocrine Surgical Oncology, Tohoku University Graduate School of Medicine, Miyagi, Japan
e-mail: takanori@med.tohoku.ac.jp

S. Nakamura
Department of Breast Surgical Oncology, Showa University School of Medicine, Tokyo, Japan
e-mail: seigonak@med.showa-u.ac.jp

T. Ohta et al. (eds.), *Practical Guide to Hereditary Breast and Ovarian Cancer III*, https://doi.org/10.1007/978-981-96-6779-6_11

genic variant carriers. Nearly 400 unaffected *BRCA1/2* pathogenic variant carriers have already been enrolled in this registry project. It is considered urgent to develop a system of medical care for unaffected *BRCA1/2* pathogenic variant carriers.

Keywords *BRCA1/2* · HBOC · Database · JOHBOC registry

11.1 Overview of JOHBOC Registry

It is estimated that 5–10% of all cancers are associated with a genetic predisposition. Two genes, *BRCA1* and *BRCA2,* are known to be highly involved in the development of breast and ovarian cancers. Pathological mutations in the *BRCA1/2* gene are associated with hereditary breast ovarian cancer (HBOC) and have an increased risk of developing certain cancers such as breast, ovarian, prostate, and pancreatic cancers compared to the general population. In recent years, *BRCA1/2* genetic testing has expanded remarkably in Japan, and after being listed as a companion diagnosis to determine the indication of olaparib, a PARP inhibitor, for patients with metastatic or recurrent breast cancer or recurrent advanced ovarian cancer in April 2018, it became partially covered for patients with breast or ovarian cancer with suspected HBOC in April 2020. At this time, risk-reducing mastectomy (RRM) and risk-reducing salpingo-oophorectomy (RRSO) for HBOC patients with a history of breast or ovarian cancer and surveillance with MRI scans were also partially covered by insurance. In January 2021, insurance coverage was extended to patients with pancreatic cancer that is not curatively resectable and metastatic castration-resistant prostate cancer as a companion diagnosis to determine the indication for olaparib and to high-risk recurrent breast cancer in 2022.

As one of its projects, the Japanese organization of hereditary breast and ovarian cancer (JOHBOC) was established in August 2016 in cooperation with the Japan Society of Human Genetics, the Japanese Breast Cancer Society, and the Japan Obstetrics and Gynecology Society, with the aim of improving and expanding the medical treatment system for HBOC and suspected HBOC patients and their families, and to contribute to the improvement of medical care and preventive medicine for the nation [1]. One of JOHBOC's main projects is a registry of hereditary breast and ovarian cancer families. The clinical and genetic characteristics of HBOC in Japan should be clarified, because there are regional and population group differences in cancer incidence. A nationwide registry of hereditary breast and ovarian cancer cases will allow us to determine the clinical and genetic characteristics of HBOC in Japan, including the characteristics of pathogenic variants of the *BRCA1/2* gene and the incidence of cancer among those who carry the pathogenic variants. In addition, by understanding the actual status of *BRCA1/2* pathogenic variant carriers in Japan through genetic testing, we will be able to offer appropriate screening, diagnosis, and treatment options to patients and their families, which may lead to a decrease in mortality rates from breast and ovarian cancers. Therefore, in the JOHBOC registration project, a database of hereditary breast and ovarian cancers has been established and participation is being solicited from medical facilities throughout Japan, with the aim of elucidating the clinical and genetic characteristics in the Japanese population and linking this to standard treatment by improving the medical environment for the parties concerned and including them in the guidelines. The participating facilities in the registry must be able to provide appropriate genetic counseling and genetic testing for eligible patients within their facilities. Information on patients and family members who have given consent using the prescribed patient explanation documents and patient consent forms in accordance with the research protocol will be registered. To establish a system for the long-term accumulation of follow-up data on registrants, registered data are updated once a year for all cases and a list of registered cases for the relevant year is made at the end of August each year for each fiscal year. For the history of the registration project to date, please refer to the previous report [2–4]. Beginning with the 2022 registry, this registry project will be open to families who have undergone *BRCA1/2* genetic testing and had a positive test result (Deleterious or Suspected Deleterious) or Variant of Unknown Significance (VUS) and who have undergone *BRCA1/2* genetic testing. The registry is divided into four categories: (1) individuals who had a *BRCA1/2* genetic testing performed at a registry facility, (2) individuals who had a *BRCA1/2* genetic testing performed at another facility and who received subsequent treatment and follow-up at a registry facility, (3) blood relatives who are registered based on information provided by the participant, and (4) others. If a participant is found to be registered in the another facility, we will contact the other institution with the consent of each participant in order to minimize duplicate registrations. In the next section, we report a summary of the September 2022 national registration data tabulation results.

11.2 Summary of JOHBOC Registration Data for 2022

11.2.1 Number of Registrations

A total of 134 facilities participated in this registration project: 3610 *BRCA1/2* pathogenic variant carriers with a history of attending these centers were enrolled (*BRCA1*: 1770, *BRCA2*: 1826, *BRCA1/2*: 14) (Table 11.1). Of these, 382 (10.6%) had no cancer at the time of genetic testing. There were 639 enrollees with VUS detected in *BRCA1/2* (*BRCA1*: 192, *BRCA2*: 440, *BRCA1/2*: 7).

11.2.2 Registered Variants

There were 359 registered pathogenic variants of the *BRCA1* gene. The variant with the highest number of reports was c.188 T > A (p.Leu63*), with 317 patients registered. This was followed by 117 registrations for c.2800C > T (p.Gln934*) and 40 for c.2389_2390del (p.Glu797Thrfs*3) (Table 11.2). There were 279 pathogenic

Table 11.1 Background of 3,610 BRCA1/2 pathogenic variant carriers enrolled in the JOHBOC registry

Item		Number of registrations	
BRCA1/2	*BRCA1*	1770	(49.0%)
	BRCA2	1826	(50.6%)
	BRCA1/2	14	(0.4%)
Gender	Female	3451	(95.6%)
	Male	159	(4.4%)
Onset of cancer	Unaffected	382	(10.6%)
	Affected	3228	(89.4%)

Table 11.2 BRCA1 pathogenic variant with the highest number of registrations in the JOHBOC registry

Exon	HGVS cDNA	HGVS protein	Number of registered cases
5	c.188T>A	p.Leu63*	317
11	c.2800C>T	p.Gln934*	117
11	c.2389_2390del	p.Glu797Thrfs*3	40
24	c.5558A>G	p.Tyr1853Cys	28
3	c.131_132del	p.Cys44*	27
19	c.5154G>T	p.Trp1718Cys	21
11	c.3442del	p.Glu1148Argfs*7	20
16	c.4964C>T	p.Ser1655Phe	20
11	c.2075_2076del	p.His692Argfs*19	19
20	c.5278-1G>A		17

Table 11.3 *BRCA2* pathogenic variant with the highest number of registrations in the JOHBOC registry

Exon	HGVS cDNA	HGVS protein	Number of registered cases
13	c.6952C>T	p.Arg2318*	181
11	c.5576_5579del	p.Ile1859Lysfs*3	152
23	c.9076C>T	p.Gln3026*	79
10	c.1813del	p.Ile605Tyrfs*9	64
20	c.8504C>A	p.Ser2835*	61
11	c.5645C>A	p.Ser1882*	59
18	c.8023A>G	p.Ile2675Val	44
23	c.9117G>A	p.Pro3039=	44
10	c.1278del	p.Asp427Thrfs*3	36
11	c.6405_6409del	p.Asn2135Lysfs*3	33

variants of the *BRCA2* gene registered. Of these, the most frequent variant was c.6952C > T (p.Arg2318*), with 181 registered. Next, c.5576_5579del (p.Ile1859Lysfs*3) was registered by 152 individuals and c.9076C > T (p.Gln3026*) by 79 individuals (Table 11.3). For VUS, 96 types were registered for the *BRCA1* gene and 138 types for the *BRCA2* gene.

11.2.3 Risk-Reducing Surgery

There were 439 *BRCA1/2* pathogenic variant carriers who underwent RRM (*BRCA1*: 234, *BRCA2*: 203, *BRCA1/2*: 2). Of these, 402 (91.6%) were contralateral RRM and 37 (8.4%) were bilateral RRM. The average age at RRM was 45.7 years. Of the 439 enrollees who underwent RRM, occult breast cancer was detected in 36 (8.2%) (*BRCA1*: 16; *BRCA2*: 20). On the other hand, 831 *BRCA1/2* pathogenic variant carriers who underwent RRSO were registered (*BRCA1*: 430, *BRCA2*:396, *BRCA1/2*: 5). The mean age at RRSO was 49.5 years. Occult ovarian cancer was detected in 14 (1.7%) of the enrollees who underwent RRSO (*BRCA1*: 9, *BRCA2*: 5).

11.2.4 Contralateral and Ipsilateral Breast Cancers

Among *BRCA1/2* pathogenic variant carriers who developed breast cancer, 499 women who underwent breast-conserving surgery were available for follow-up after the genetic testing. Of these, ten ipsilateral breast cancers were observed after the genetic testing (Table 11.4). On the other hand, there were 1339 women with unilateral breast cancer and *BRCA1/2* pathogenic variants who were available for follow-up after genetic testing. Of these, 72 developed contralateral breast cancer after the genetic testing (Table 11.5).

11.2.5 *Unaffected* BRCA1/2 *Pathogenic Variant Carriers*

There were 366 unaffected *BRCA1/2* pathogenic variant carriers (64 males and 302 females) who could be followed after genetic testing. The mean age at which a genetic testing was performed was 44.4 (24–72) years for men and 40.0 (18–82) years for women. The mean observation period after the genetic testing was 0.8 years (0–13.1) for men and 2.0 years (0–20.8) for women. During the observation period,

Table 11.4 Ipsilateral breast cancers in *BRCA1/2* pathogenic variant carriers

	BRCA1	*BRCA2*	*BRCA1/2*
Breast-conserving surgery cases (Traceable cases)	242 cases	254 cases	3 cases
Ipsilateral breast cancer after the genetic testing	7 cases	3 cases	0 cases
Observation period after the genetic testing (mean, median)	0.1–14.3 years (1.9, 0.9)	0.1–18.1 years (1.9, 0.7)	0.1–1.4 years (0.7, 0.8)
Background			
Age at first onset of breast cancer (in years) (Average)	23–80 (41.9 years)	19–75 (45.6 years)	38–55 (45.0 years)

Table 11.5 Contralateral breast cancer in *BRCA1/2* pathogenic variant carriers

	BRCA1	*BRCA2*	*BRCA1/2*
Unilateral breast cancer incidence (traceable cases)	585 cases	750 cases	4 cases
Contralateral breast cancer after genetic testing	33 cases	38 cases	1 case
Observation period after the genetic testing (mean, median)	0.1–20.0 years (1.8, 0.9)	0.1 to 22.4 years (1.8, 0.7)	0.1–13.0 years (5.0, 3.5)
Background			
Age at first onset of breast cancer (in years) (Average)	23–84 (43.2 years)	19–80 (44.4 years)	34–78 (53.8 years)

Table 11.6 List of proposals adopted for 2022 (6th JOHBOC national registration)

Research themes	First presenters	Affiliated institutions
Examination of the association between the status of a desire to undergo CRRM and patient background factors	Chika Sato	Kansai Medical University
Clinicopathological Features of Non-invasive Ductal Carcinoma of breast in the Japanese HBOC Cohort - Comparison with Invasive Ductal Carcinoma of breast	Dai Kitagawa	National Center for Global Health and Medicine
Breast Cancer Risk Reduction Strategies for Previously Diagnosed Ovarian Cancer Patients with *BRCA1/2* pathogenic variant	Junko Minato	Tohoku University Hospital

2 of the men developed other cancers, 47 of the women developed breast cancer, 6 developed ovarian cancer, and 5 developed other cancers.

11.3 Research Issues Using Data from the JOHBOC Registry

In this registry project, the goal is to use the database to publish articles or present at academic conferences to deliver new knowledge to medical professionals. For clinical research proposals, we invite applications once a year from participating institutions that meet certain criteria, such as registration of follow-up data, and select about two to three proposals per year by designating research themes and first presenters based on discussions at the registry committee. The adopted proposals are to be presented at a scientific meeting sponsored by JOHBOC and published. Several proposals are currently in progress, and Table 11.6 shows the three newly adopted research proposals for 2022 (the sixth national registration). Other requests for clinical research using the database and thc usc of data as a control for clinical research at an institution are also accepted at any time.

11.4 Future Outlook

In this registry project until 2020, when *BRCA1/2* genetic testing for breast and ovarian cancer patients with suspected HBOC was covered by insurance, more than half of the *BRCA1/2* pathogenic variant carriers were *BRCA1* pathogenic variant carriers [4]. However, in the current tally, more than half of the patients were *BRCA2* pathogenic variant carriers. The number of examinees has increased as the financial burden on examinees has been reduced, and it is thought that the number of examinees has come to reflect the situation in Japan, which is closer to the actual situation. Since the input system in this registry project has established a system that can accumulate follow-up data of registrants over a long period of time, it is expected to provide more accurate and useful information for *BRCA1/2* pathogenic variant carriers in Japan. In addition, an input system was established to allow more detailed registration of information on prostate cancer and pancreatic cancers starting in 2024. It is expected that data on these cancers as well as breast and ovarian cancers will be accumulated in the future. However, the HBOC care system in our country currently does not cover *BRCA1/2* genetic testing, risk-reducing surgery, and appropriate surveillance for unaffected *BRCA1/2* pathogenic variant carriers. In this registry project, nearly 400 unaffected *BRCA1/2* pathogenic variant carriers have already been registered, and there is an urgent need to improve the medical treatment system for these patients.

Acknowledgments JOHBOC Registration Committee: [Committee]:Arisa Ueki (Cancer Institute Hospital), Yoshinori Akama (Tochigi Cancer Center), Hiroki Den (Showa University), Narumi Harada (Tohoku University), Takeo Kosaka (Keio University), Hiraku Kumamaru (Tokyo University), Chigusa Morizane (National Cancer Center Hospital), Masato Ozaka (Cancer Institute Hospital), Ayumi Shikama (Tsukuba University), Kanae Taruno (Showa Univerity). [Secretariat of JOHBOC]: Eriko Shimamoto. Participating 134 institutions that entered their data with our 2022 registry: Aichi Cancer Center Hospital, Aichi Medical University Hospital, Akita University Hospital, Aomori Prefectural Central Hospital, Asahikawa Medical University, Cancer Institute Hospital, Chiba University, Ehime University, Fujisawa City Hospital, Fujita Medical University, Fukui Prefectural Hospital, Fukui University, Fukuoka University Hospital, Fukuoka Wajiro Hospital, Fukushima Medical University, Gifu University, Gunma Prefectural Cancer Center, Hamamatsu Medical Center, Hamamatsu University School of Medicine, University Hospital, Hiroshima Prefectural Hospital, Hiroshima University, Hokkaido Cancer Center, Hokkaido University, Hoshi General Hospital, Hyogo Cancer Center, Hyogo Medical University, Hyogo Prefectural Amagasaki General Medical Center, Ibaraki Prefectural Hospital, Ishikawa Prefectural Central Hospital, Iwate Medical University, JA Hiroshima General Hospital, JA Onimichi General Hospital, Japan Community Health care Organization Sagamino Hospital, Japanese Red Cross Aichi Medical Center Nagoya Daini Hospital, Japanese Red Cross Ishinomaki Hospital, Japanese Red Cross Medical Center, Japanese Red Cross Nagoya Daiichi Hospital, Japanese Red Cross Saitama Hospital, Japanese Red Cross Yamaguchi Hospital, Jisenkai Aizawa Hospital, Juntendo University, Kagawa Prefectural Central Hospital, Kagawa University Hospital, Kagoshima University Hospital, Kanagawa Cancer Center, Kanazawa Medical University Hospital, Kanazawa University, Kansai Electric Power Hospital, Kansai Medical University, Kato Breast Surgery Clinic, Kawasaki Medical School, Keio University, Kindai University Hospital, Kitano Hospital,

Kitazato University, Kochi Medical Center, Kochi University, Kokura Medical Center, Kyoto City Hospital, Kyoto Miniren Chuo Hospital, Kyoto University, Matsue City Hospital, Matsue Red Cross Hospital, Matsushita Memorial Hospital, Medical Journal of Japanese Red Cross Society Wakayama Medical Center, Mie University Hospital, Nagasaki University, Nagoya City University, Nagoya Ekisaikai Hospital, Nagoya University, Nara Prefecture General Medical Center, National Center for Global Health and Medicine, National Hospital Organization Kyoto Medical Center, National Hospital Organization Kyushu Medical Center, National Hospital Organization Osaka National Hospital, Nihonkai General Hospital, Niigata University, Nippon Medical School, Nishiwaki Municipal Hospital, Ogaki Municipal Hospital, Oikawa Hospital, Okayama University, Okazaki City Hospital, Osaka General Hospital of West Japan Railway Company, Osaka International Cancer Institute, Osaka Metropolitan University Hospital, Osaka Police Hospital, Osaka Red Cross Hospital, Osaka University, Osaki Citizen Hospital, Sagara Hospital Breast Center, Saiseikai Hyogoken Hospital, Saitama Medical University International Medical Center, Sapporo Medical University, Sapporo Tokushukai Hospital, Seirei Hamamatsu General Hospital, Sekishindo Hospital, Shikoku Cancer Center, Shikoku Medical Center for Children and Adults, Shinshu University, Shiroyama Hospital, Shizuoka Cancer Center, Shizuoka General Hospital, Shizuoka municipal Hospital, Shonan Memorial Hospital, Showa University Hospital, Showa University Koto Toyosu Hospital, St. Lukes Hospital, St. Marianna University School of Medicine, Suwa Red Cross Hospital, The Jikei University, Tohoku University Hospital, Tokushima University Hospital, Tokuyama Central Hospital, Tokyo Medical Center, Tokyo Metropolitan Komagome Hospital, Tokyo Saiseikai Central Hospital, Toranomon Hospital, Tosei General Hospital, Tottori Prefectural Central Hospital, Tottori University, Toyama Prefectural Central Hospital, Toyama University Hospital, Toyohashi Municipal Hospital, Toyota Memorial Hospital, University of Miyazaki Hospital, University of Tsukuba, University Of Yamanashi Hospital, Yamagata Prefectural Central Hospital, Yamaguchi Rosai Hospital, Yamaguchi University, Yamanashi Prefectural Central Hospital, Yokohama City University, Yokohama City University Medical Center.

References

1. Japan Hereditary Breast Cancer Ovarian Cancer Comprehensive Medical Care System Organization. https://johboc.jp/. Accessed 29 Feb 2024.
2. Arai M, Yokoyama S, Watanabe C, et al. Genetic and clinical characteristics in Japanese hereditary breast and ovarian cancer: first report after establishment of HBOC registration system in Japan. J Hum Gent. 2018;63(4):447–57.
3. Arai M, The Registration Committee of the Japanese Organization of Hereditary Breast and Ovarian Cancer (JOHBOC). Hereditary breast and ovarian cancer. Hereditary Breast and Ovarian Cancer (HBOC) database in Japan. In: Nakamura S, Aoki D, Miki Y, editors. Hereditary breast and ovarian cancer molecular mechanism and clinical practice. Singapore: Springer; 2021. p. 243–57.
4. Inuzuka M, Arai M, Nakamura S. Registration data of Japanese Organization of Hereditary Breast and Ovarian Cancer till 2020. In: Aoki D, Nakamura S, Miki Y, editors. Practical guide to hereditary breast and ovarian cancer annual meeting of the Japanese Organization of Hereditary Breast and Ovarian Cancer 2021. Singapore: Springer; 2023. p. 145–54.

MIX
Papier aus verantwortungsvollen Quellen
Paper from responsible sources
FSC® C105338

If you have any concerns about our products,
you can contact us on
ProductSafety@springernature.com

In case Publisher is established outside the EU,
the EU authorized representative is:
Springer Nature Customer Service Center GmbH
Europaplatz 3, 69115 Heidelberg, Germany

Printed by Libri Plureos GmbH
in Hamburg, Germany